Applied Psychology in Health Care

Applied Psychology in Health Care

Donnie J. Wilbanks, MA, BA

Instructor, Psychology and Anatomy and Physiology
St. Louis College of Health Careers
St. Louis, Missouri

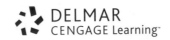

DELMAR
CENGAGE Learning

Australia • Brazil • Japan • Korea • Mexico • Singapore • Spain • United Kingdom • United States

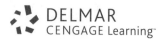

Applied Psychology in Health Care
Donnie J. Wilbanks

Vice President, Career and Professional Editorial: Dave Garza

Director of Learning Solutions: Matthew Kane

Acquisitions Editor: Matthew Seeley

Managing Editor: Marah Bellegarde

Senior Product Manager: Debra Myette-Flis

Editorial Assistant: Megan Tarquinio

Vice President, Career and Professional Marketing: Jennifer McAvey

Marketing Manager: Michele McTighe

Marketing Coordinator: Scott Chrysler

Production Director: Carolyn Miller

Content Project Manager: Anne Sherman

For product information and technology assistance, contact us at
Professional & Career Group Customer Support, 1-800-648-7450

For permission to use material from this text or product, submit all request online at **cengage.com/permissions**. Further permissions questions can be e-mailed to **permissionrequest@cengage.com**.

Library of Congress Control Number: 2008925996

ISBN-13: 978-1-4180-5348-2

ISBN-10: 1-4180-5348-1

Delmar
5 Maxwell Drive
Clifton Park, NY 12065-2919
USA

Cengage Learning products are represented in Canada by Nelson Education, Ltd.

For your lifelong learning solutions, visit **delmar.cengage.com**

Visit our corporate website at **cengage.com**.

Notice to the Reader

Publisher does not warrant or guarantee any of the products described herein or perform any independent analysis in connection with any of the product information contained herein. Publisher does not assume, and expressly disclaims, any obligation to obtain and include information other than that provided to it by the manufacturer. The reader is expressly warned to consider and adopt all safety precautions that might be indicated by the activities described herein and to avoid all potential hazards. By following the instructions contained herein, the reader willingly assumes all risks in connection with such instructions. The publisher makes no representations or warranties of any kind, including but not limited to, the warranties of fitness for particular purpose or merchantability, nor are any such representations implied with respect to the material set forth herein, and the publisher takes no responsibility with respect to such material. The publisher shall not be liable for any special, consequential, or exemplary damages resulting, in whole or part, from the readers' use of, or reliance upon, this material.

Printed in the United States of America
1 2 3 4 5 6 7 XX 12 11 10 09 08

Contents

Preface

The field of health care contains many diverse disciplines. Institutions that educate and train students in these disciplines do a good job of delivering programs of instruction that provide the knowledge and skills required. This is, of course, necessary; but it does not thoroughly prepare the student for a career in health care. Skill only matters if you can apply it and health care is applied in a relationship. After students graduate and embark on their careers the two elements that all of the very different disciplines have in common are the health care provider and the client. The nature of their relationship can enhance the quality and effect of the care given and the patient's compliance with that care, or it can detract from that quality and possibly generate noncompliance. It must be remembered that in the end, health care is not a technical but a human enterprise. Quality health care requires the active participation of everyone involved—the provider, the client, the family, sometimes even the friend. Fact-based knowledge and skills create ability, but ability must be balanced with information that helps providers to better understand themselves and their clients. Psychology applied to health care must provide an overview of psychology that helps the provider better understand their own development and functioning, allows them to recognize and challenge their own beliefs and biases, and provides them with a better understanding of clients and their often perplexing and sometimes hostile behavior.

The first goal of vocational psychology is to provide the student with a general understanding of the forces and processes that mold personality and influence behavior. Understanding that there are reasons for the things we and others do is a necessary first step in learning to accept both ourselves and others.

The second goal of vocational psychology is to place the student's own beliefs in perspective. After they complete their education, health care students will provide a wide range of services. In today's aging, actively mobile, ever-changing, multicultural environment, health care providers must frequently supply services to patients whose practices and beliefs they may not fully understand or appreciate. Gaining an understanding of their own beliefs and identifying their own biases will help them develop the ability to withstand the stresses of caregiving, suspend judgment, and act professionally.

The final goal of vocational psychology is to familiarize the future health care provider with issues that will likely affect their client's emotions and behaviors.

Bias, stress, loss, and grief can all create difficult emotions and behaviors, and mental illness affects a much larger percentage of clients than is normally recognized (Silverstone, 1996; Friedman, 1997). A fuller understanding of all of these issues and of their impact on the client can enable the provider to better accept and aid clients as they struggle to cope and adjust.

For over five years I searched for a psychology text that would provide material for these goals in a concise form that could be taught in a one semester course. My inability to locate that text has led to the development of this book.

This text is intended primarily for vocational allied health students. This includes licensed practical nurses, patient-care technicians, medical assistants, certified nursing assistants, massage therapists, pharmacy technicians, medical billing and coding personnel, X-ray technicians, EKG technicians, and many other specialties. I believe it would also be applicable in registered nurse, physical therapist, occupational therapist, speech therapist, and respiratory therapist training, and other similar programs. Additionally, due to its general approach to human understanding, I believe it would be helpful to anyone involved in a helping relationship, whether as a helper, or as a client.

ORGANIZATION OF THE TEXT

The text is divided into three broad sections: "Psychology," "The Provider," and "The Client." The "Psychology" section provides the theoretical foundation. The first chapter in this section begins with a discussion of the physical foundation of behavior. This foundation involves the influences of genetics and the environment as they apply to the development of the nervous system and the structural and functional divisions of the brain. The chapter ends with a discussion of the nature of consciousness. The second chapter explores the development of personality. It presents a model of psychological functioning, and within this framework discusses needs, feelings, beliefs, and behaviors, and culminates in a description of personality traits. The third chapter explores culture, community, and parenting styles as they influence the development of personality, and the final chapter looks at psychological function, dysfunction, adjustment, change, and the effects of stress.

The "Provider" section contains three chapters. The first focuses on recognizing our own beliefs and overcoming the effects of bias and discrimination. The second chapter considers the role of the caregiver, discusses professionalism, and more deeply explores a set of skills that can be practiced and developed to enhance the provider's caretaking ability. The final chapter of this section discusses professional ethics, the client-provider relationship, client rights, and provider responsibilities.

The third section, "The Client," begins with a discussion of loss and grief, the types of each, explores grieving behavior, and continues with an exploration of the issues that affect clients as they seek medical care. These issues include adjustment to loss, irrational beliefs, and mental illness. The chapter ends with an overview of the categories and types of mental illness.

Following the body of each chapter is a brief summary of the major ideas presented and a review of each important concept in the order they appear within the chapter. This concept review is intended to serve as a study guide for the student.

FEATURES OF THIS BOOK

There are many features of *Applied Psychology in Health Care* designed specifically to enhance the student's comprehension of the material.

- **Objectives** help guide the student through important concepts to be learned.
- **Key Terms** are boldfaced when defined in the text. A comprehensive **glossary** is included in the back of the book.
- **Application Skill** feature encourages students to deepen their understanding of "soft" skills introduced in the chapter through real-world situations.
- **Chapter Summary** emphasizes the main points of the chapter.
- **Concept Review** serves as a study guide of each important concept in the chapter.

- **Review Questions** help students to assess their comprehension of the chapter material.
- **Critical Thinking Questions** promote a broader understanding of key points.

Application Skill Feature

To be useful, vocational psychology must not only provide a deeper understanding of ourselves and others, it must also provide an ability to apply that understanding in the provision of health care. The application sections at the beginning and end of each chapter in this book will be used to present a set of skills to accomplish that purpose. A skill is an ability that can be learned to more effectively accomplish a purpose. Nursing and allied health schools teach specific sets of "hard" skills, such as taking a blood pressure or making a nursing assessment. Knowledge of these hard skills is what separates medical assistants from patient care technicians, pharmacy technicians, and so on. But there are also "soft" skills such as listening and communication that can be applied in every area of specialization to improve health care at all levels. These "soft," or human, skills are used to look at and truly see, listen to, and communicate with patients; to resolve patient issues; and, finally, to help health care providers control themselves in stressful situations. These skills include: observation, active listening, assertiveness, communication, relaxation, anger management, non-defensiveness, encouragement, problem-solving, and behavioral modification.

FOR THE INSTRUCTOR

The requirement for teaching general education courses such as psychology, mathematics, ethics, or communication in a vocational setting is often an earned degree that contains one class in the subject to be taught. Instructors teaching such courses are seldom professionals in that field, and sometimes have taken only that one class in the subject area. I have taught courses under those conditions and have found my needs to be simple and basic: a general understanding of what the student should be getting out of each chapter, a brief overview of the material to be covered, a detailed lesson plan to guide the lecture, and test options to evaluate the results. The Instructor's Manual that accompanies this text makes provision for each of these needs. It is my hope that those teaching this course will find it concise and useful.

THE ELECTRONIC CLASSROOM MANAGER

ISBN 1-4180-5349-X

The Electronic Classroom Manager is a robust, computerized tool for all your instructional needs. A must-have for all instructors, this comprehensive and convenient CD-ROM contains the following:

- **The Instructor's Manual** is designed to help you with lesson preparation and performance assessment. It includes answers to review exercises in the text.
- **Exam View® Computerized Testbank** contains over 350 questions. You can use these questions, and add your own questions, to create review materials or tests.
- **PowerPoint® Presentations** are designed to aid you in planning your class presentations. If a student misses a class, a print-out of the slides for a lecture makes a helpful review page.

ABOUT THE AUTHOR

Following high school and service in the United States Marine Corps, the author received a BA in Behavioral Science from Missouri Baptist College and an MA in Social

Science from Webster University in St. Louis, Missouri. The author has worked as a Southern Baptist minister; alcoholism counselor; union business agent; Missouri Children's Services (child abuse) social worker; and as an in-home family therapist, compiling 18 years of social work and counseling experience. From 1998 to the present, the author has been a member of the faculty at St. Louis College of Health Careers where he has primarily taught anatomy and physiology and psychology, but has also taught mathematics, communications, ethics, sociology, medical terminology, and professional development. He provides counseling services to the students, and at times to the faculty of the college. He has been named Instructor of the Quarter and Instructor of the Year; received the outstanding service award; and was listed in 2007 and 2008 in *Who's Who in America* and in *Who's Who Among Executives and Professionals*.

REVIEWERS

We wish to thank the following instructors for their comments:

MaryAnn Edelman, MS, CNS, RN
Assistant Professor
Department of Nursing
Kingsborough Community College
Brooklyn, New York

Connie Rockstad, RN, MSN
Director of Nursing Program
Whatcom Community College
Bellingham, Washington

Mary Gormandy White, MA
Co-Founder
Mobile Technical Institute
Mobile, Alabama

Section 1
Psychology

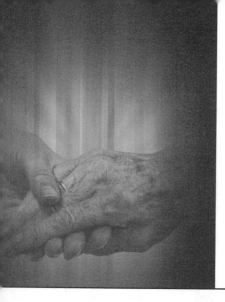

Chapter 1

Upon completion of this chapter you should be able to:

1. Define DNA.
2. List the three divisions of the nervous system and describe the function of each.
3. Describe and discuss the subdivisions of the motor nervous system.
4. Name the working cells of the nervous system and describe their basic structure.
5. Define synapse.
6. Define neurotransmitter and neuroinhibitor and explain the function of each.
7. Define and list the steps of neurodevelopment.
8. Describe how neurons make decisions.
9. Discuss the function of astrocytes.
10. Describe the anatomical structure of the brain.
11. Explain the functional divisions of the brain.
12. Discuss consciousness.

KEY TERMS

DNA	apoptosis	limbic system
fraternal twins	necrosis	neocortex
identical twins	skills	consciousness
neurons	summation	void
synapse	astrocytes	metaphysics
neurotransmitters	fight-or-flight reactions	
neuroinhibitors	reptilian complex	

The Physical Foundation of Behavior

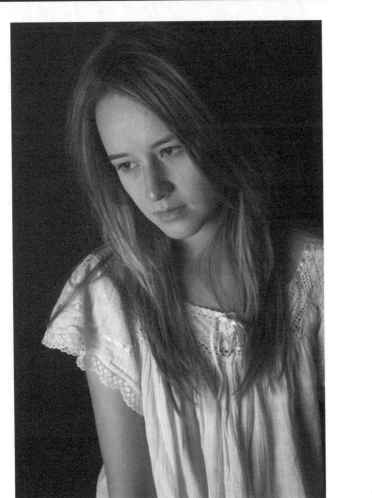

Look

You enter a room to meet a patient for the first time. She sits with her head down, eyes pointed toward the floor. As you cross the room, what do you already know about her?

INTRODUCTION

This chapter is about the physical structure that creates behavior. That structure is the nervous system and this section looks at how it develops, its parts and pieces, how it works, what it allows us to do, and the factors that influence how it grows.

Look for how decisions are made, how our behavior is affected by the genetic material we inherit from our parents, and for the many ways that interactions with our environment mold the development and functioning of our brain.

After studying this section you should have a basic knowledge of the structure and function of the nervous system and the brain and a deeper understanding of the factors that cause us to become who we are and to do what we do.

NATURE VERSUS NURTURE

Why do we humans do the things we do? We are the most aggressive and ruthless, and at the same time the most generous and caring species on earth. In the past fifteen hundred years genocide has been happening somewhere on the planet ninety-seven percent of the time. Over thirty million men, women, and children have been killed in the name of ethnic cleansing. In the twenty-five years between 1975 and 1999 there were ninety-five wars. Yet during that same time countless lives have been saved and made better by the millions who have devoted their lives in hospitals and schools, nursing homes and soup kitchens, or simply by unselfishly being there when someone needed them. We are a puzzle. Why do we do the things we do? Is it as simple as some are born good and others bad? In the era of kings and lords it was taken for granted that breeding (who your parents were) created character, which produced behavior. A few hundred years later, while behavioral psychology was at the height of its influence, it seemed clear that behavior was produced solely by rewards in the environment. Now it seems that both sides were right. Human behavior is the product of traits inherited from your mother and father in the DNA they provided, and of the brain's response to the environment you are raised in. To understand behavior you must understand the effects of heredity and environment, nature and nurture.

THE INFLUENCE OF DNA

Nature begins with **DNA**, which is an amazingly complex set of plans (genes) stored in the nucleus of each of our cells that provides the information for building and running our bodies. We receive half of these plans from our mother and half from our father, delivered in the egg and the sperm that began our lives. Brothers and sisters have 50% of their genes in common. This is also true for **fraternal twins**, who develop from separate eggs and are simply brothers or sisters with the same birthday. But **identical twins** develop from one fertilized egg and so have identical DNA. Our DNA is our heredity, so if heredity determines behavior, identical twins should behave identically. They do not. Each has a distinct identity, so obviously behavior is not completely decided by our genes. But there can be remarkable similarities. Again we are left wondering. Are the similarities the result of their identical DNA or of having been raised together at the same age in the same environment? Is it possible to separate the effects of heredity from the effects of the environment? It may be. When identical twins are separated at birth the effects of environment are minimized because similarities cannot be attributed to being raised in the same family, or sometimes even in the same town. In these situations an opportunity is created to assess how much of what we do is determined not by our environment, but by our genes.

One such set of twins was separated when they were four weeks old and raised in separate cities with no knowledge of, or contact with, each other. When they were reunited at 39 years of age they were both deputy sheriffs; drove the same model of blue Chevrolet; owned dogs named Toy, one pure white, the other pure black; they chain-smoked the same brand of cigarettes; both had the same hobby—woodworking; and both had gone to the same beach in Florida on vacation. When given personality tests they were very similar on traits of self-control, flexibility, and sociability (Leo, 1987).

While such remarkable similarities were not true for every set of separated twins studied, the consistency of unexplained similarities found demonstrates that our genes indeed play a large role in determining what we do (Bouchard, et al., 1990; Bouchard, 1994). Our genes exert this influence because they are the plans for constructing and running the most complex biological structure known, the human nervous system.

THE NERVOUS SYSTEM

Imagine you are in a large building, locked in a room without doors or windows. You have no way to know what is happening in the rest of the building, or in the world outside, and no way to affect anything beyond the room you are in. But if switches were installed on all of the doors of the building and connected by wires to lights on a display in the room, one light for each door, if a door were opened you would know because its light would glow on the board. You could install an array of devices: cameras, microphones, sensors for pressure, temperature, wind, and humidity, and so on that would enable you to gather a wide range of information about the world outside of your room. You could also install controls in the room wired to mechanical devices that would allow you to open or close, lock or unlock doors; move things around; change the temperature; and in dozens of other ways interact with the world outside of your room.

The nervous system is much the same. The brain is locked away inside of the skull. In order to know anything about the world outside, information must be brought in. Wires are connected to sensors that bring a wide range of information from your eyes, ears, nose, tongue, skin, tendons, and internal organs to your brain. Controls in your brain are connected by more wires to devices (muscles and glands) that enable you to move, walk, talk, and in general respond to and act on the world around you.

Neurons

The cells that make all of this possible are **neurons** (Figure 1.1). Each neuron has three basic parts: the cell body is the bulk of the cell and contains the nucleus and the rest of the machinery; dendrites are fibers that carry electrical impulses to the cell body;

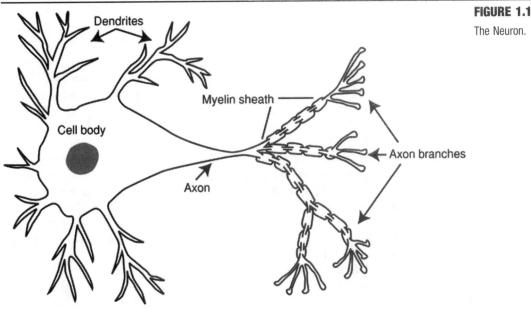

FIGURE 1.1

The Neuron.

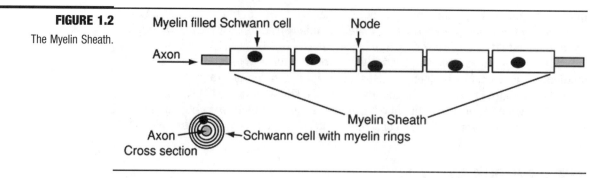

FIGURE 1.2

The Myelin Sheath.

and axons are fibers that take electrical impulses away from the cell body. Dendrites and axons run together as tracts, which are long bundles of fibers that connect neurons to each other inside of the brain and spinal cord (central nervous system), and as nerves, which are such bundles outside of the brain and spinal cord (peripheral nervous system). The dendrites and axons of tracts and nerves are like wires that conduct electrical currents to and from the neurons. A current is a flow of something. Just as a river current is a flow of water, an electrical current is a flow of charged (electromagnetic) particles. The electricity that lights our houses is a flow of negatively charged particles called electrons. Our nervous system uses positively charged sodium ions (Na+) and potassium ions (K+) flowing along nerve fibers—dendrites and axons—to relay information.

The Myelin Sheath

Dendrites and axons are small around but can be very long, some connecting your toes to your spinal cord. Sodium and potassium ions are tiny, so it takes time for them to flow over this great a distance; too much time to allow the nervous system to operate efficiently. It would be like turning on a light to read by and having it come on some time tomorrow. To speed-up the process, specialized cells flatten out a fat—cholesterol—like a pancake and wrap it around some of the fibers. This creates the myelin sheath (Figure 1.2).

When a fiber is wrapped in the myelin sheath the ions do not flow through the entire length of the fiber, but rather skip from one node to the next. This is called salutatory conduction and it is an extremely fast way to conduct electrical impulses.

Synapse

To receive and pass on information, neurons in the brain grow a web of connections with each other. Each has from tens of thousands to over a hundred thousand connections with other neurons (Figure 1.3), and each of these connections is a highly specialized structure called a **synapse** (Figure 1.4).

An electrical impulse sent out from a neuron travels along one of its axons until it forms a synapse (connection) with another neuron. The cells do not ever actually touch. There is always a space between them. To transmit an electrical impulse to the second neuron the axon releases chemicals called **neurotransmitters** into the cleft (space) between them. These neurotransmitters have the ability to start the flow of ions, an electrical impulse, on the second neuron. This is the way a neuron says "yes."

A neuron also has the ability to release chemicals that make it harder for an impulse to be generated on the second neuron. These chemicals are **neuroinhibitors**. This is the way a neuron says "no."

The key to the nervous system lies in the complex interactions between neurotransmitters and neuroinhibitors in the vast network of *one hundred billion neurons* that make up the brain and spinal cord. While a computer has one processor, and handles one piece of information at a time, the neurons create millions to billions of

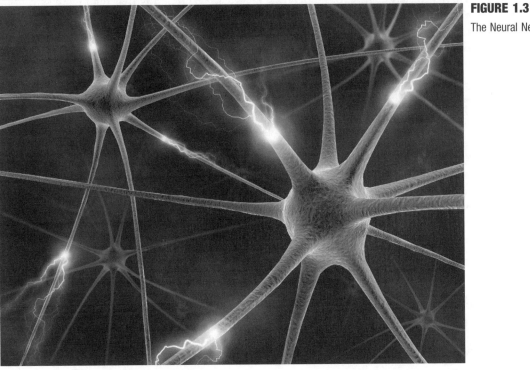

FIGURE 1.3

The Neural Network.

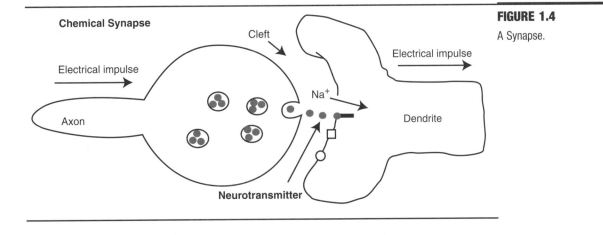

FIGURE 1.4

A Synapse.

parallel processors, all working at the same time, each handling a different task. Together they carry out a multitude of tasks simultaneously, each neuron making its own decisions and sending out transmitters or inhibitors by way of connecting axons in order to pass those decisions on. A neuron's ability to effectively do its job depends on the connections it makes, sometimes over one hundred thousand of them, through which it gains the input necessary to make accurate decisions.

THE INFLUENCE OF THE ENVIRONMENT

Try getting and keeping ten people organized. It takes constant attention. Now think of efficiently organizing one hundred billion neurons from a single fertilized egg. The development of the brain is a project of preposterous proportions. About 60 percent of the genes in our DNA are dedicated to it. The process begins at conception and, like the rest of the body, the brain has a lot of growing to do when the baby is born. This is natural with newborns of just about every animal species, but in humans it is at its most extreme. At birth the human brain is only about 15 percent developed.

There are two factors that make this necessary. The first is that the changes in bone structure necessary to stand upright and walk on two legs decreases the size of the birth canal. The second is that the mature human brain is enormous compared to the brains of other animals our size. In order to make birth possible at all, babies had to be born at earlier and earlier stages of development. Compared to the year or so it takes a baby to walk, a horse is following its mother around within an hour of its birth.

The fact that most of our brain development takes place after we are born creates a vast potential for adaptability. Most of a horse's brain is developing while it is still safely tucked away inside of its mother. That does not allow its brain to be shaped by its environment. The human brain is shaped directly by the environment. After a baby is born, neurons that are stimulated by interactions with the world thrive and grow the connections needed to do what is being asked of them. Neurons that are not stimulated by interactions wither away and die. This process creates a brain that is literally molded by the world it lives in, resulting in an adult perfectly in tune with that world. While most species can survive in only a very limited habitat and will become extinct if that habitat is destroyed, with the exception of the oceans or the poles, humans successfully inhabit just about every area of the earth. Adaptability is the key to our success and the ability of our brain to literally be molded to fit the world we live in, whatever that world may be, is a major factor in our adaptability.

Neurodevelopment

Before their eyes opened a group of newborn kittens was placed in an artificial environment with no vertical lines. After their eyes opened they were kept there for less than a week and then placed in a normal environment. The kittens grew up to be normal in every way except that they were completely blind to any vertical line (Lewin, 1974). The neurons that would have learned to recognize vertical lines and put them into the picture of vision were not exposed to them during a critical time frame, so they did not develop the ability to perform that task; and for the rest of their lives the cats ran headlong into table legs and chair legs. Asking neurons to perform a particular task sets in motion a process of development that creates the ability to do that task. This process creates the nervous system.

The first step in creating a functional nervous system is the creation of neurons. This is pretty much completed in the first six months of pregnancy, with extremely little production of neurons taking place beyond that age. For all practical purposes, children are born with all of the neurons they will ever have. From that point, we lose neurons for the rest of our lives. This creates a planned obsolescence. The brain of an elderly person is significantly smaller and lighter than the brain of a young person and ultimately, even if the body does not, the brain will fail.

Neurons are created with the potential to perform any task, but capable of performing none. Just as it is hard to do office work at the gym or run laps in the office, there are positions in the brain from which it is easier to make the connections needed to perform a specific task. In order to gain the ability to perform a job well, the neurons must first get into the right positions. Before birth, the positioning of neurons is directed entirely by our genes, but after birth, this migration is strongly influenced by what tasks the environment asks neurons to perform (Rakic, 1981; Rakic, 1996). Once the neurons migrate to a specific area they begin to specialize and become dedicated to one task.

The neurons that are not used do not develop. In fact, they are programmed to die. This type of cell death is called **apoptosis** and it does not cause inflammation the way unplanned cell death, caused by disease or injury and called **necrosis**, does. This is all part of the molding process. If a neuron isn't needed there is no reason for that neuron to exist, and very soon, it does not. It withers, dies, and is reabsorbed (Kuan, Roth, Flavell, & Radic, 2000).

Neurons that continue to be used begin branching: growing tree-like dendrites to connect with all of the other neurons they will need information from in order to make informed and accurate decisions. They also grow axon branches to pass those decisions on. The more a neuron is used, the more dendrite and axon branches it grows (Diamond, Law, Rhodes, et al., 1966; Greenough, Volkmar, & Juraska, 1973).

These neurons then begin connecting: forming the connections they will need with other neurons. The more a neuron is used, the more connections it will make. This process continues throughout life, with new connections being formed as new knowledge or **skills** are learned. The junctions that continue to be used regularly are enlarged, strengthened, and bound more closely and securely together. They become much more efficient at quickly transmitting impulses. Synapses that cease to be used break down and the axons degenerate (Huttenlocker, 1994).

The final step in the development of neural pathways is production of the myelin sheath. Pathways that are used regularly are sheathed soonest, and when the process is completed it greatly speeds the conduction of impulses and makes many things, like walking, possible.

Many of these key processes in the development of the brain are dependent on the experiences of the developing child. Without the appropriate environmental cues—being talked to, cuddled, played with, stimulated, and so on—the brain cells are not capable of appropriately organizing and maturing (Lauder, 1988; Perry, 1994; Perry & Pollard, 1998).

DECISIONS

Thousands of connections can bring in an enormous amount of information. Each input from another neuron comes in the form of a neurotransmitter, which serves to excite the neuron and cause it to generate an electrical impulse, or a neuroinhibitor, which acts to prevent an electrical impulse from being generated. Whether or not an electrical impulse is actually generated depends on the combined effect of all of the neurotransmitters and neuroinhibitors from all of the other neurons with which a neuron is connected. This is called **summation**, and it is a democratic decision. If the neurons saying "yes" outnumber the ones saying "no" by a large enough margin, an electrical impulse is generated.

Astrocytes

This democratic process of summation is modified by another set of brain cells that actually outnumber the neurons; these are the astrocytes. **Astrocytes** do not make decisions themselves, but send out arms that surround and engulf some of the synapses in a specific group of neurons. A group of neurons connected by an astrocyte is called a domain (Figure 1.5).

An astrocyte has the ability to override the normal neurotransmitter/neuroinhibitor balance and generate impulses on all of the neurons in its domain simultaneously (Cornell-Bell, Finkbeiner, Cooper, 1990). They tie a related group of neurons together and cause them to operate as one unit, thereby coordinating brain activity. The astrocytes are attracted to the junctions (synapses) between neurons that are the most frequently used (Cornell-Bell, Thomas, Caffrey, 1992); they strengthen these connections, drawing the ends closer together. If connections cease to be used, the astrocytes pull back and the neuron is isolated. Isolated neurons are used much less, so in time the neuron's connections are broken down, the fibers withdrawn, and the neuron can be reabsorbed. The effect of this is to coordinate and strengthen functions that are used and eliminate functions that are not used.

ORGANIZATION OF THE NERVOUS SYSTEM

As the nervous system develops, neurons specialize and form themselves into three functional divisions. The three divisions of the nervous system are made of sensory, association, and motor neurons (Figure 1.6).

FIGURE 1.5

An Astrocyte Domain.

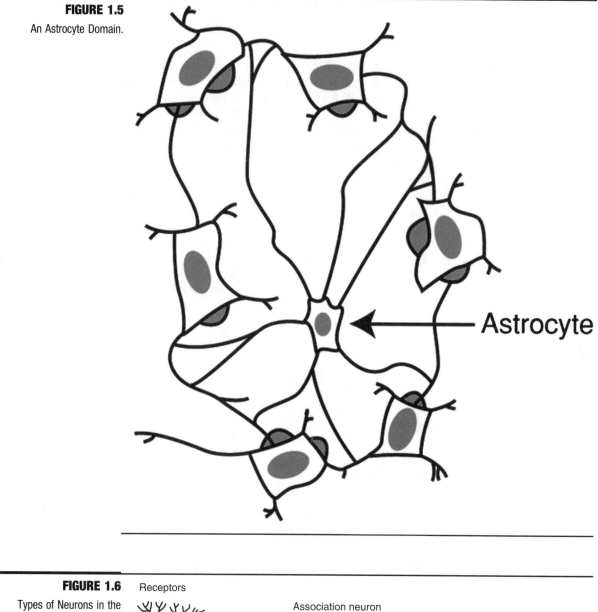

Astrocyte

FIGURE 1.6

Types of Neurons in the Nervous System.

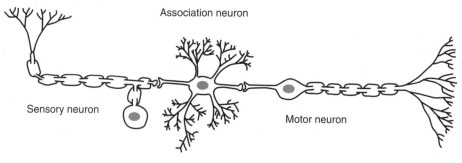

Receptors

Association neuron

Sensory neuron

Motor neuron

The Sensory Division

The cell bodies of the sensory neurons move just outside of the brain or spinal cord and extend fibers far into the body to pick up information and bring it to the brain or spinal cord. At the far end of these fibers is one or more receptor. This is a structure designed to start an electrical impulse when it comes into contact with one specific stimulus. There are receptors for vision, taste, smell, hearing, equilibrium, pain, skin sensation, and so on. Each receptor is essentially a switch that is turned on by

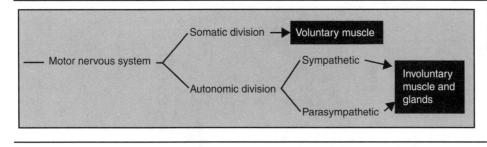

FIGURE 1.7

Divisions of the Motor Nervous System.

something in the environment, and the sensory neuron is the wire that carries the resulting electrical signal to an area in the brain designed specifically to recognize and process that information.

The Association Division

These brain areas are the home of the association neurons, which receive information from the sensory neurons and a wide array of other sources within the brain and spinal cord. They process all of this input, make decisions, and pass those decisions on to the third group, the motor neurons.

The Motor Division

Motor neurons grow fibers out of the brain or spinal cord to carry impulses back to the muscles, organs, and glands of the body, which are called effectors. The motor division of the nervous system is divided and subdivided several times. (Figure 1.7).

The primary separation splits the motor nervous system into the somatic and autonomic divisions. The somatic division carries instructions to voluntary muscles, muscles you can move at will that are attached to the skeleton and that move your body. The autonomic division carries instructions to involuntary muscles in the heart, internal organs, and blood vessels, and to glands. The autonomic division is then subdivided into sympathetic and parasympathetic sections. The sympathetic division of the motor nervous system moves things away from normal and is responsible for **fight-or-flight reactions**. These are emergency or stress responses during which the heart beats faster and harder; the blood supply to the heart and to voluntary (skeletal) muscle increases; the blood supply to digestion decreases; breathing becomes faster and deeper; sweating increases; and glucose is made readily available for energy production. The parasympathetic division of the motor nervous system returns everything to normal.

The brain and spinal cord together form the central nervous system. The sensory and motor divisions, which are made of neurons with structures at least partially outside of the brain or spinal cord, make up the peripheral nervous system.

THE BRAIN

The central processing unit for the nervous system is the great collection of tools we call the brain (Figure 1.8).

The brain has four major structural divisions; the brain stem, diencephalon, cerebellum, and cerebrum.

The Brain Stem

The spinal cord travels upward through the vertebral column to an opening in the base of the skull. As soon as it passes through that opening it becomes the brain stem. The brain stem has vital centers that control the heart rate, the rate and depth of breathing, and the flow of blood and blood pressure into the different areas of the

FIGURE 1.8

The Brain.

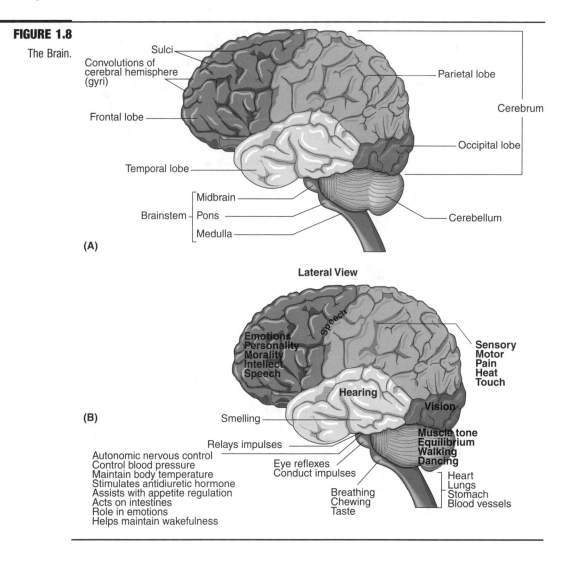

(A)

(B)

body. It also contains reflex control centers for coughing, sneezing, hiccupping, swallowing, and vomiting and for hearing and eye reflexes. It connects the spinal cord to the cerebellum and the diencephalon.

The Diencephalon

The diencephalon contains the very significant thalamus and hypothalamus. Neurons in the thalamus are connected to the spinal cord, cerebellum, and virtually every area of the cerebrum and together they act as the central relay station, deciding where incoming information needs to go and sending it there. The thalamus also produces conscious awareness of touch, pain, and temperature, as well as pleasure and alertness.

The hypothalamus is involved in a vast array of functions. It controls the body's autonomic (automatic) internal processes and produces the body's physical responses to emotional and mental states, and thus has the ability to produce psychosomatic (psycho = mind, soma = body) illness and healing. The hypothalamus also directs the endocrine system, through which it affects the functioning of every cell in the body. In addition, it is essential in maintaining a waking (alert) state; controls hunger and fullness; and regulates and maintains body temperature.

The Cerebellum

The cerebellum coordinates muscular activity. It monitors sensory input on its way from the muscles to the cerebrum and motor impulses on the way from the cerebrum to the muscles. With this information it compares the movement intended by the cerebrum with the movement the motor impulses would actually produce and sends correcting impulses to both the cerebrum and the muscles, thus coordinating muscle activity for smoother, more efficient movements.

The Cerebrum

The cerebrum is the largest part of the brain and lies over the top of almost everything else. It is divided into a section on the right and one on the left, each known as a hemisphere. Visible on the surface of each hemisphere is a frontal, parietal, temporal, and occipital lobe. The cerebrum contains sensory areas for touch, pressure, temperature, body position, vision, hearing, taste, smell, and balance as well as the motor areas for all of the muscles of the body that can be moved at will. It is also the seat of intelligence and provides memory and creativity; the ability to read, speak, write, understand higher mathematics, abstract reasoning, and music; and has centers that activate and inhibit behavior.

THE FUNCTIONAL BRAIN

As well as dividing the brain by structure, a useful way to think of the brain is as being divided into functional layers. The functional layers of the brain are the stem, the reptilian complex, the limbic system, and the neocortex (Sagan, 1977) (Figure 1.9).

These functional layers of the brain are arranged with the most primitive structure, the brain stem, at the base; then the reptilian complex; followed by the limbic system; and finally the most complex structure, the neocortex, at the top. Each unit has its own job to do, its own needs to meet. These needs create feelings, which drive behaviors designed to meet the needs. The higher the brain layer, the more complex its needs and the more complex are the feelings and the behaviors designed to meet them.

The Brain Stem

The brain stem is the most primitive part of the brain and takes care of processes vital to physical survival. The brain of a fish is composed entirely of a brain stem, and anything a fish is capable of can be done with one. But if you want to be smarter than a fish and interact with the world in more complex ways, you need a more complex brain. Since you are depending on the brain stem to keep you alive, you can't simply discard it and start over; you have to build a more complex layer over it, while allowing the brain stem to continue to do its job. The next most complex layer of the brain is the reptilian complex.

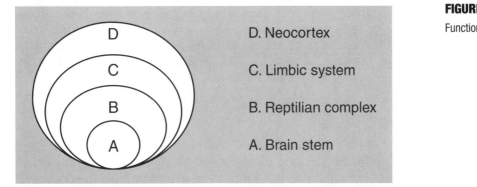

FIGURE 1.9

Functional Brain Divisions.

Reptilian Complex

As the name implies, the **reptilian complex** is found in the brain of reptiles. It is the seat of status and territory and drives the ritual and aggression by which status and territory are protected and maintained. In nature, status is created by power. The larger, faster, more powerful control the best territory, and territory provides food, water, and shelter, all of the necessities of life. The territory controlled by the smaller, slower, weaker provides less of the necessities of life. When looking for a potential mate, a female is attracted to the male who controls the territory that will provide the best chance for the survival of her offspring. Others who are allowed entry into the territory defer to the one who controls it. In my life my territory is composed of the people and things that provide for my needs. My wife, children, and family; my country, home, the area I live in; my position, job, career; and my friends—these are all part of my territory and I depend on them. The better my territory is able to provide for my needs, and the better my territory is able to provide for the needs of others, the higher my status will be and the more I will be deferred to. I will defend my territory and my status within my territory against any who threaten them, first with ritual warning displays of facial expression, body language, tone of voice, and words, and if these are not sufficient, with verbal or physical aggression.

Limbic System

The limbic system is the next layer, more complicated than the reptilian complex, designed to allow us to interact in still more complex ways. It is sometimes called the mammalian complex, because it separates the brain of a reptile from the brain of a mammal. The **limbic system** is a ring of structures at the base of the cerebrum that is known as the emotional brain. Behaviors arising from this level include the sexual and social behaviors that bring us together and make it possible for us to live in cooperative groups. The ability to understand and use logic also develops here, but it is concrete, working only as a means to get what is wanted or avoid what is not wanted.

The Neocortex

The **neocortex** is the most complex layer of the brain. It is composed of the bulk of the cerebrum, and it powers abstract thought, essential for the concepts involved in ethics, morals, philosophy, mathematics, and strategy. This is the level that creates the characteristics that we identify as "human." It provides us with the ability to conceive of something that we "ought" to do to and pushes behavior to achieve that.

CONSCIOUSNESS

Consciousness is the greatest mystery of all. Everything that has been discussed so far could be reasonably well duplicated, at extremely great trouble and expense, by technology. But no one would expect the resulting hardware to be self-aware. We are very complicated biochemical machines and like any machine in many ways we are merely the sum of our parts. If something goes wrong with a part, the machine breaks down. We are also more than that, and we are not sure why. What is it about the machinery that creates consciousness?

The Spirit

For much of history consciousness has been equated with the spirit. Though there have been and are still many beliefs, the spirit has generally been seen as nonmaterial, eternal, intelligent, motivating, and conscious; the body without the spirit as lifeless, decomposing, and unconscious; and life without the expression of spirit as slow, dull, unmotivated—uninspired. The origin of belief in a spirit is unknown, but the belief itself is extremely widespread and is the basis of most religion.

Chemical Consciousness

Exactly what consciousness is remains illusive, but we can certainly see what affects it. Currently the dominant scientific view involves concentrations of neurotransmitters and the organization and activity of neurons. Consciousness depends on continual impulses to the cerebrum from a formation of cells in the brain stem called the reticular activating system. Waking up in the morning depends on increased activation by this system and without its constant impulses a person is unconscious and cannot be aroused. Barbiturates decrease alertness and produce sleep by depressing the activity of the reticular activating system. Local anesthesia involves blocking the transmission of sensory impulses from a specific location. Some general anesthetics, which produce unconsciousness, may work by completely blocking the flow of the chemicals responsible for sensory impulses.

Quantum Consciousness

An emerging, but controversial, concept of consciousness is quantum consciousness (Mendel, 2000). In order to understand the concepts involved, it is first necessary to grasp some basics of quantum mechanics. As this is being described remember that this is not fantasy or speculation, though many have believed it to be. Albert Einstein found quantum mechanics so difficult to accept that he spent much time and effort attempting to disprove it. Quantum mechanics, or quantum physics, is the mathematics and science that deals with the particles that make up atoms. Since all the matter in the universe is made of atoms, everything in the universe is made of these particles. But these particles follow a completely different set of rules than the atoms they create. Atoms obey classical physics, which describes how solid particles in the universe act and interact. The particles that make up atoms obey quantum physics. Classical physics and quantum physics are so different that the two do not overlap. Predictions made by one system about the other are ridiculous.

Atoms and the matter they make exist as real objects in the universe; the particles that make them up exist as waves of probability, quantum waves, in the void. Everything that exists has this dual nature, existing simultaneously as a particle in the universe and as a quantum wave in the void. So, what is the void?

The Void

It is hard to describe what the **void** is because time, space, matter, energy, and all the other things of the universe do not exist in the void the same way they exist here. Time does not exist there, everything happens at once. Space does not exist; everything is in all possible places at all times. Cause and effect can reverse, with the effect appearing before the cause. Time can reverse, with the future appearing before the past. Our current language and logic are inadequate to describe this kind of reality; we need a new understanding, a new logic, and a new language. Mathematics is currently the only language that describes the void, but this has all of the character of describing a flock of birds in flight by plotting their variable speeds and positions.

The void is first and foremost power. Power is the ability to bring about a state of real existence rather than possibility. Power creates possibility and then brings it into real existence as a particle in this universe by shaping it with the law of probability. Following this law possibilities interact to become probabilities, and probabilities interact to become realities.

Probability is the likelihood of becoming real. When probabilities interact they can interfere with each other and become weaker, or they can combine and become more powerful until they grow into a wave of probability, a quantum wave, powerful enough to emerge with an objective, independent existence in the universe.

It becomes a solid, real particle in the universe, while at the same time maintaining its existence in the void. Every particle has this dual nature. It exists as a particle in the universe, and as a quantum wave in the void. As a particle in the universe it obeys one or more of the four forces: gravity, electromagnetism, the strong force, and the weak force. As a quantum wave it obeys the law of probability.

There is reason for speculation that consciousness exists in quantum waves isolated in our brain. The charges on the ions flowing along a neuron are electromagnetic. One understanding of consciousness is that as positively charged particles flow into a neuron from a dendrite they attract the negatively charged electrons on the microtubules that make the skeleton of the cell, and reposition them. The quantum waves of these electrons interact with pure quantum waves isolated inside of the microtubules, so when they are repositioned this feeds information into the quantum waves. Consciousness may be an interpretation, or awareness, in the quantum wave of incoming impulses. Unconsciousness results from interfering with these incoming electrical impulses, blocking the quantum wave's access to and awareness of the information.

Quantum Computers

If this is true we should be able to duplicate it. By learning to use electromagnetism to feed information into quantum waves, quantum computers have been developed. The potential is staggering. Computers with a processing unit handle one piece of information at a time; but time doesn't really exist in the quantum wave. By a process called superposition, every possible reality exists simultaneously there. In the void everything happens at once. Quantum computers have the potential to be vastly more powerful than a conventional computer. Even though they are still very rudimentary, by establishing that information can be stored and retrieved, and decisions made, in quantum waves, quantum computers support the possibility that consciousness may be a quantum phenomenon.

The mind's activity demonstrates many of the characteristics of quantum waves. Abstract thinking and intuition do not resemble the A + B = C simple logic of a normal computer; they demonstrate the superposition, logic, and reversals of the void.

Quantum consciousness contains elements of both spiritual and chemical consciousness. It relies on the flow of chemicals arriving at neurons, so an interruption of the flow of those chemicals will affect it. It also relies on unknown, and perhaps unknowable, processes carried out in the void.

Metaphysics

Metaphysics has traditionally described the existence of a realm where time, space, and matter do not exist, yet which is the source of all that exists in the universe. It is much more of a philosophy than a science but it is common to both science and religion. The difference is that science sees the power there as one *that* creates and sustains the universe. Most religions see the power there as one *who* creates and sustains the universe.

SUMMARY

An amazing amount of what we do is determined by our DNA, the genetic material we received from our parents. These are plans, called genes, for making and running our bodies. Over 60 percent of them are for growing and running the brain and the brain directs our behavior. But when we are born the brain is only about 15 percent developed, and completing its growth is a long and complex process that requires both genetic plans and interactions with the environment. The working cells of the brain are neurons. At birth most neurons are immature and incapable of functioning. When a baby first interacts with the environment the brain is asked to see, hear, understand, direct the body, and so on; things it cannot yet do. But asking it to do them begins the process of developing the neurons and gaining those abilities. The more often the brain is asked to do a thing the faster and better it grows the connections between neurons it takes to do it. Our DNA moves us through distinct developmental stages during which interactions with the environment shape the brain's inner structure at each level. The developed brain may be divided both structurally and functionally, and each area is responsible for its own tasks. Taken together these tasks enable us to be aware of what is going on in the world around us and respond to it in amazingly complex ways. Perhaps the most complex achievement of the brain is consciousness itself. There are many conceptions of consciousness; just what it is remains illusive, but it seems possible that it exists in a realm that is beyond our language, our understanding, and even our concepts.

APPLICATION SKILL

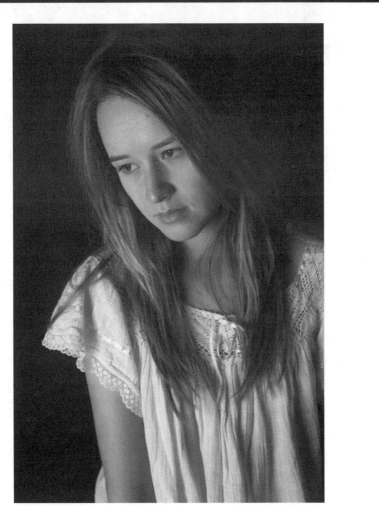

Look

You enter a room to meet a patient for the first time. She sits with her head down, eyes pointed toward the floor. As you cross the room, what do you already know about her?

The primary human skill is looking. As simple as that may sound, many people do not look at each other. There are many reasons: some consider it to be rude; others see it as a challenge or an insult; some are shy or unsure; and many are just distracted by their own thoughts or concerns. Whatever the reasons for not looking, the reasons for looking are compelling. Looking at others is our primary method of gathering information about them. Human DNA provides a plan for the construction of an extensive information-processing

APPLICATION SKILL *(continued)*

apparatus in the brain that almost instantly interprets a wealth of information about another person. Facial expression and coloration; body position and posture; arm position; eye contact and content; clothing—not just what is worn but how it is worn; grooming; and much more. All of the pieces are combined into patterns until they emerge in us as an intuitive feeling that tells us how and sometimes whether to approach a person. To gather and reason through all of that information could take hours or days, but it is all available in the time it takes to walk across a room and say hello. Do not glance at a patient, look at them. See them. Many specialties in health care teach specific observational skills, but Mother Nature has endowed us with an innate ability that can provide a foundation stone for every other skill we may possess. All we have to do to access that ability is to look.

CONCEPT REVIEW

DNA – The genetic material inside of cells that contains the plans for making and running the body.

stimulus-response – The nervous system allows us to recognize what is going on in the world around us and respond to it.

neurons – The working cells of the nervous system that conduct electrical impulses and make decisions.

dendrites – Fibers that carry electrical impulses to the neuron cell body.

axons – Fibers that carry electrical impulses away from the neuron cell body.

cell body – The bulk of the neuron, contains the DNA and cell machinery.

central nervous system – The brain and spinal cord.

peripheral nervous system – All the nervous tissue outside of the brain and spinal cord.

tracts – Long bundles of nerve fibers that carry electrical impulses inside of the central nervous system.

nerves – Long bundles of nerve fibers that carry electrical impulses in the peripheral nervous system.

myelin sheath – A covering wrapped around some nerve fibers that greatly increases the speed of electrical impulses.

synapse – A specialized structure that forms a junction between two neurons or between a neuron and another type of cell. This structure is capable of passing the electrical impulse across a gap from one cell to the next. A neuron usually has thousands and sometimes more than a hundred thousand connections with other neurons.

neurotransmitters – Chemicals that pass an electrical impulse from one neuron to another across a synapse.

neuroinhibitors – Chemicals that stop electrical impulses from being passed from one neuron to another across a synapse.

neurodevelopment – The growth and organization of the nervous system. Without interaction with the environment much of this development does not take place, or if it has taken place, the connections and neurons quickly degenerate.

decisions – All of the neurons with which one neuron is connected have input into the decisions the neuron makes. A neuron says to another neuron, "yes, do that," by sending one or more neurotransmitters to it across a synapse. A neuron says to another neuron, "no, don't do that," by sending one or more neuroinhibitors to it across a synapse. If a neuron receives more neurotransmitters than neuroinhibitors from the other neurons with which it is connected it generates an electrical impulse.

astrocytes – Support cells in the brain and spinal cord that tie a group of neurons together by sending out extensions that surround the synapses connecting the neurons with each other. They are attracted to the synapses that are used the most.

domain – A group of neurons tied together by one astrocyte. An astrocyte has the ability to override the normal neurotransmitter/neuroinhibitor balance and cause all of the neurons in its domain to generate electrical impulses at the same time. Synapses and neurons that are used too little can degenerate, wither, and die. The effect of this process is to speed and strengthen functions that are used and eliminate functions that are not used.

divisions of nervous system – The nervous system has three primary divisions made up of three types of neurons; sensory, association, and motor.

sensory neurons – A sensory neuron begins with a receptor somewhere in the body. The receptor is a switch that can be turned on by a change in the environment. When the switch is turned on an electrical current (impulse) travels through the sensory neuron and into the brain or spinal cord, where it sends neurotransmitters through a synapse to an association neuron.

association neurons – The association neuron receives the neurotransmitters from the sensory neuron and from multiple other association neurons and makes a decision. It relays this decision to a motor neuron by sending neurotransmitters through a synapse.

motor neurons – Motor neurons receive electrical impulses from association neurons and take the impulse out into the body to an effector—a muscle or a gland.

motor nervous system – The motor neurons are divided into two groups, the somatic and the autonomic divisions.

somatic – Motor neurons that carry electrical impulses to voluntary muscles, muscle that can be moved at will.

autonomic – Motor neurons that take electrical impulses to glands and to involuntary muscle in the heart, organs, and blood vessels. The autonomic nervous system is subdivided into the sympathetic and the parasympathetic divisions.

sympathetic division of the autonomic nervous system – Motor neurons that conduct impulses that move the functioning of the endocrine glands, heart, organs, and blood vessels away from normal. The sympathetic division is responsible for fight-or-flight and stress reactions.

parasympathetic division of the autonomic nervous system – Motor neurons that conduct impulses that return the functions of the endocrine glands, heart, organs, and blood vessels back to normal.

brain – Encased in the skull the brain is the central processing unit for electrical impulses coming in from sensory neurons and going out by motor neurons. It may be divided by structure and what that structure enables the body to do, and by function and how that function allows the person to interact with the environment.

structural divisions of the brain – Structurally the brain is divided into the brain stem, the diencephalon, the cerebellum, and the cerebrum.

brain stem – The brain stem carries out processes vital to the physical well being and survival of the body. It connects the rest of the brain to the spinal cord.

cerebellum – The cerebellum coordinates the activities of voluntary muscle.

diencephalon – The diencephalon contains the thalamus and the hypothalamus and is the major switchboard of the brain, sending all impulses to their proper locations. It is also responsible for the body's automatic physical processes and for the mind-body connection.

cerebrum – The cerebrum is the largest part of the brain and is responsible for awareness of physical sensations, voluntary responses, and sight. It is the seat of higher mental functions such as creativity, art, analytical thinking, and mathematics; and it contains the behavior activation and behavior inhibition centers.

behavior activation center – The association area in the cerebrum that assumes that behavior will be successful and causes actions to be performed.

behavior inhibition center – The association area in the cerebrum that assumes that behavior will not be successful, initiates doubt, and stops behavior from being performed.

functional divisions of the brain – Functionally the brain may be divided into the brain stem, the reptilian complex, the limbic system, and the neocortex.

brain stem – The most primitive structure in the brain the stem forms its central core and controls processes vital to the physical functioning of the body.

reptilian complex – The layer of the brain immediately over the brain stem. The reptilian complex enables more complicated behavior by establishing perception of status (one's position relative to others) and how we interact with others based on that perception.

limbic system – Developed after the reptilian complex, the limbic system motivates and guides group behavior by facilitating emotion, memory, and motivation.

neocortex – The latest and most complex development in the brain, the neocortex is responsible for the higher mental functions that we identify with being human and humane.

consciousness – Awareness, including self-awareness.

spirit – Historically, consciousness has been explained as a spirit living within us.

chemical consciousness. – The contemporary scientific view is that consciousness is the result of patterns and concentrations of neurotransmitters (chemicals) in the brain.

quantum consciousness – An emerging view of consciousness as awareness based in quantum waves isolated in the neurons of the brain. Quantum consciousness contains elements of both spiritual and chemical consciousness.

metaphysics – Reality and rules beyond the limits of our universe and our understanding. Science and religion both recognize the existence of this reality.

science – Identifies metaphysics as an existence and a power *that* creates and sustains the universe.

religion – Identifies metaphysics as an existence and a power *who* creates and sustains the universe.

REVIEW QUESTIONS

I.   Completion

Complete the following sentences.

1. _____ is the genetic material inside of the nucleus of cells that contains the plans for making and running the body.

2. The brain and spinal cord together make up the _____ nervous system.

3. What determines the number of dendrites and axons an association neuron grows to connect with other neurons? _____.

4. A neuron says to another neuron, "yes, do that" by sending _____ across the synapse. It says "no, don't do that" by sending _____ across the synapse.

5. The contemporary scientific view of consciousness sees it as arising from patterns and concentrations of _____ in the brain.

II.   Multiple Choice

Select the letter of the choice that best completes the statement.

6. A section of the DNA that contains a set of plans for one specific physical trait.
   A. Chromosome
   B. Nucleic acid
   C. Codon
   D. Gene

7. Fibers that carry electrical impulses to the cell body of the neuron.
   A. Axon
   B. Dendrite
   C. Myelin
   D. Synapse

8. Nerve impulses carried along nerve fibers are actually a flow of
   A. Positively charged ions
   B. Negatively charged ions
   C. Electrons
   D. Electricity

9. A covering wrapped around some nerve fibers that greatly speeds up electrical impulses.
   A. Axon
   B. Dendrite
   C. Myelin
   D. Synapse

10. The fate of neurons that are not asked to perform a task or that cease to be used.
    A. Apoptosis
    B. Necrosis
    C. Boredom
    D. Migration

III.   Matching

Match each term with its correct description.

   A. Environment
   B. Synapse
   C. Identical twins
   D. Astrocyte
   E. Peripheral nervous system

_____ Develop from one egg and have the same DNA.

_____ All the nervous tissue outside of the brain and spinal cord.

_____ A specialized structure connecting two neurons.

_____ The immediate world we live in and respond to.

_____ Causes all of the neurons in its domain to work as one functional group.

IV.   Critical Thinking

11. How does an individual's DNA determine his or her behavior?

12. How does an individual's environment determine his or her behavior?

13. What is the purpose of the nervous system?

14. Why can neurons be described as democratic?

15. Why is the structure of each adult's brain different from the structure of any other?

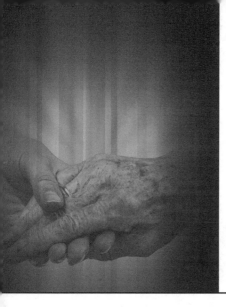

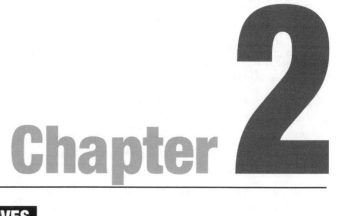

Chapter 2

CHAPTER OBJECTIVES

Upon completion of this chapter you should be able to:

1. Define personality.
2. Name and define the four stages of cognitive development.
3. Describe the model of psychological functioning and define each step.
4. List and define the needs in Maslow's hierarchy.
5. List and define Kohlberg's moral levels.
6. List and define the stages of emotional development.
7. List and define each trait of the five trait personality theory.
8. Describe the dynamics of personality development.

KEY TERMS

personality	emotions	extraversion
cognitive stages	actions	agreeableness
psychological model	behavior	conscientious
needs	moral levels	neuroticism
feelings	emotional development	openness to experience
self-talk	personality traits	

The Development of Personality

APPLICATION SKILL

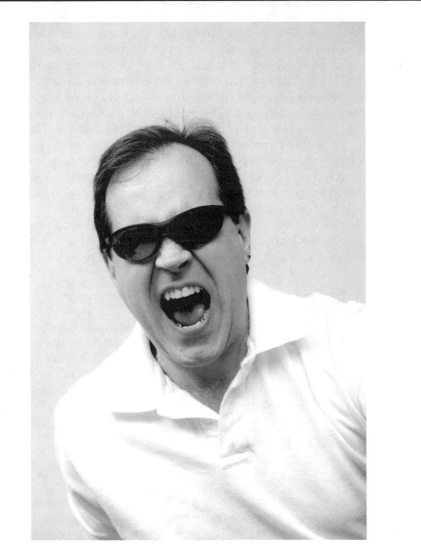

Wait

Using the skill of really looking at the client, what is your reaction to the person you see in this photograph? If you had to deal with him how do you think you would approach him? What do you think you would feel?

INTRODUCTION

This chapter defines personality and describes the process of personality development. It introduces a model of psychological functioning that will be used throughout the rest of this book.

Look for the psychological model, Maslow's hierarchy of needs, Erikson's emotional dilemmas, and the five traits of personality.

After studying this chapter you should be familiar with each step of the psychological model proposed. You should have a basic knowledge of the factors involved in the development of personality and of the five trait personality theory.

PERSONALITY

People everywhere have much in common. We are after all, all human. But no one is exactly like anyone else. When we get to know someone we recognize that person as a distinct individual. If we know them well we come to know what to expect from them, how they will react, what they will think about or say about something. We know if we can depend on them; if they will understand or accept what we have done; if they will try something new; if they will initiate the conversation or if we need to approach them; if they will see the good in the situation, or dwell on the negative. Each of us has a character, that is, a set of characteristics that is stable over the years and from one situation to the next. That set of stable characteristics is our **personality**, which is a set of traits that begins with genetic plans and is completed as those plans are expressed by physical growth in the brain as it develops in response to the demands of the environment. This brain growth is carried out in a series of steps called cognitive stages that allow the child time to work through stages of emotional development and learn sets of beliefs, emotions, and actions to meet a succession of progressively more complex needs. The outcome of this development is a set of personality traits that are consistent over time in different situations and that define the individual's engagement with others throughout his or her lifetime. The goal of this process is to produce adults capable of negotiating their world well enough to survive, develop friendships and associations, mate, and protect and nurture their young. These are the skills required for a species to survive on earth, and the success of the species is built on individuals successfully learning to meet their own needs.

COGNITIVE STAGES

Part of the genetic heritage we share as humans is a staged process of brain development. Children are not asked to sort out everything at once; rather they go through a series of stages that are focused on specific developmental tasks, and for which abilities develop one set at a time. This gives them time to experience their world and learn simple tasks before moving on to more complex functions later. Jean Piaget described a series of four **cognitive stages** from infancy to adulthood (Roth et al., 2000).

Stages of Cognitive Development

Sensorimotor

For about the first two years of life feelings created by sensory input (hunger, cold, etc.) lead directly to motor (physical) responses with little complex processing. The needs that drive behavior are largely physical. The child responds to direct interactions with the parent, physical and material power, reward and punishment.

Symbolic Functions

From about two to seven years of age the ability to create and maintain mental images and symbols and to express them as language develops rapidly. Children learn and use self-advancing bargains and compromises to stay safe and secure and to get what they want or avoid what they don't want. The child is self-centered, with very little ability to see the world from any viewpoint other than their own.

Concrete Functions

Between the ages of about seven to eleven years logic and reason develop and are used in a black or white manner, dealing with what is present in the moment in order to gain what is wanted or avoid what is not wanted. Approval, affection, and acceptance are sought from those holding power in the family, and in the group. Sexuality develops.

Formal Operations

After about age twelve, or beginning at puberty, higher mental functions requiring abstract thought emerge. The ability to understand and use principles, think through alternatives, and base behavior on beliefs of what should be develops. Needs for recognition and respect from others grow into the need for self-respect, requiring motivation and direction from within.

PSYCHOLOGICAL MODEL

We emerge from this staged developmental process with a set of traits in place that give us the ability to interpret the world and respond to it in a consistent, organized manner. To understand how these traits develop and how they affect us we need to put them into the context of how we function emotionally and psychologically. To see this clearly we need a **psychological model** (Figure 2.1).

Needs

Needs are the things we require to survive and live a normal life. We need food, water, air, and pressure. We need to be safe and secure. We need to receive and give love, affection, and acceptance. We need to belong, first in a family, and then to go beyond the family and be accepted in a group. We need respect and self-respect, and finally, we need to be able to be truly ourselves, to be motivated and directed from within. It is the brain's job to keep track of whether we have enough of all of these things and if we don't to somehow get us to do something about that. If we stop breathing carbon dioxide builds up in our blood stream. That information is relayed to the brain over sensory nerves and the brain takes action, creating neurotransmitters that start an electrical signal flowing along motor nerves leading to the muscles we breathe with, causing them to contract, pulling air into our lungs. This is a basic physical process taken care of by the most basic part of the brain, the brain stem. At a higher level the limbic system takes care of emotional needs such as love and belonging. If we don't

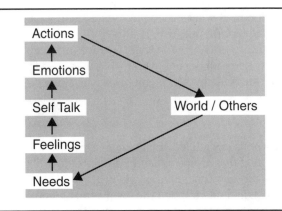

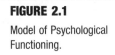

FIGURE 2.1

Model of Psychological Functioning.

have enough of one of these it is the limbic system's job to get us to do something about that. But what we have to do to get love or acceptance is far more complicated than getting muscles to contract to pull air into our lungs. More complex needs require more complex processing and more complicated actions, so the unconscious part of our brain enlists the help of the part of our brain that is conscious and has access to these higher-level skills. It does this in the only way neurons have to communicate: it produces neurotransmitters and sends them across synapses to other brain cells. These neurotransmitters create feelings. Under normal conditions, it does us no good to feel a need when there is no possibility of meeting it, so the unconscious mind keeps track of the gradual increase of a need and of the external situation. When a situation arises that makes it possible for the need to be met, neurotransmitters are released which create a conscious awareness of the need. This is a feeling and it drives us to take some action to meet the need. If a situation that provides the opportunity for the need to be met does not arise, or if our actions are not successful in getting the need met, the need grows stronger. If it grows strong enough powerful feelings can be generated which drive us to find a way to meet the need in inappropriate situations.

Feelings

Feelings are the unconscious mind's way of communicating needs to the conscious mind. Hunger tells us we need to eat; loneliness tells us to do something about not having enough love, or acceptance. Feelings tell us that we need, but they can't tell us what to do to fill that need. We have to learn what to do, but people and situations change—what we learned to do to be accepted in grade school most likely won't work in college or on the job. We need a set of rules that are consistent over time and from one situation to the next to keep us stable by helping us interpret the present situation and decide what action to take. These rules are our beliefs. We form a system of beliefs about ourselves, others, the world, and often about God. These beliefs are not always conscious, we may not be aware of them, but they affect us in powerful ways just the same. The key to understanding them is to listen to what we are saying to ourselves, to our self-talk.

Self-Talk

We process the who, what, when, and where of every situation with beliefs, which are often deep and unspoken, about ourselves, about other people, and about the world in general. This results in powerful self-statements, **self-talk**, which reflect our appraisal of the situation. This appraisal includes the set of emotions and actions (behaviors) that we anticipate will most likely succeed in getting what we need out of this situation. This appraisal transforms our feelings into emotions.

Emotions

Emotions are feelings that have been molded by the appraisal reflected in our self-talk. "He really doesn't understand what he's doing" leads us in a completely different direction than "He's doing that on purpose, just to spite me." One statement turns irritation into tolerance, the other can end in rage. One feeling can potentially be molded into any number of emotions, all depending on what we are saying to ourselves about the situation. Self-talk turns feelings into emotions, emotions power actions.

Actions

Actions are physical responses such as eating, facial expressions, body language, talking, walking, and listening that are designed to affect the world or other people (pull air into your lungs, take food into your stomach, bring a person into your life) in such a way as to meet the original need. When the need is met a new round of neurotransmitters is produced, creating a feeling of satisfaction that stops the action.

In summary, the unconscious part of the brain detects a lack of some element necessary for an individual to survive, develop friendships and associations, mate, protect and nurture their young, or to be fully themselves. This lack is a need and it is communicated to the conscious part of the brain by way of neurotransmitters that create a feeling. The individual processes this feeling along with other information such as the who, what, when, and where of the situation, with established beliefs about self, others, and the nature of the world. These suggest probable outcomes of potential actions. These are encapsulated into self-talk, which reflects the person's appraisal of all of the elements of the situation and which changes the feeling into an emotion. The emotion powers an action. Together the emotion and action comprise **behavior**. The goal of the behavior is to meet the need by getting the element necessary to relieve the original lack, enabling individuals to survive, develop friendships and associations, mate, protect and nurture their young, or to be true to their own nature. Meeting the need results in the production of neurotransmitters, which create feelings of contentment, pleasure, and so on that remove the motivation to act.

MASLOW'S HIERARCHY OF NEEDS

Surviving is about meeting needs, and learning to thrive is about learning how to meet more and more complicated needs well. This is far too complex to do all at once, so the brain moves through stages of development, each in turn devoted to interacting with the environment and learning behaviors to meet ever more complex needs. An American psychologist, Abraham Maslow, described these needs as a hierarchy, meaning that we move through them one step at a time from the least to the most complex (Maslow, 1970). The lowest need that is chronically unmet will grow larger and more insistent until it dominates the person's feelings, thoughts, emotions, and actions. Stop breathing for three minutes and see how concerned you are about anything other than getting another breath of air. This hierarchy can be illustrated in a stair-step arrangement (Figure 2.2).

Needs

Physical needs are the basic needs and they are easy to identify; if they aren't met well enough, you die. They include air, food, water, warmth, and pressure. If these needs are not met they quickly grow to dominate behavior, centering the person around the effort to meet the need and relieve the distress. Safety and security is more complicated. If you are unsafe you may not die, but you are in danger of harm

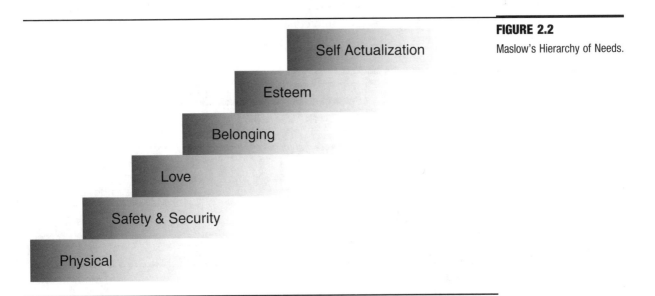

FIGURE 2.2

Maslow's Hierarchy of Needs.

Self Actualization

Esteem

Belonging

Love

Safety & Security

Physical

or death. Security is the feeling of being able to stay safe, and it depends on learning to understand your environment and developing the ability to negotiate it well enough to believe yourself capable of avoiding harm. Love is acceptance, appreciation, and affection from one or a few important individuals in your life. Belonging is acceptance and inclusion; it begins in the family and then extends out of the family into a group. Esteem is recognition and respect first from others in the group, and then from your self. Self-actualization is motivation and direction from within, being guided by your own principles and your own conscience.

Moral Levels

Maslow's hierarchy establishes multiple levels of needs that must be met in order. Over time the lowest-level need that is consistently unmet grows ever more powerful until it motivates thoughts, emotions, and actions at that level. This motivation is the key to what Lawrence Kohlberg (1984) termed moral levels. **Moral levels** are defined not by what we do, but by why we do it. As the lowest order need that is chronically unmet grows powerful it motivates behavior that can most often be defined and predicted by the morals at that level. Moral levels can be correlated with the unmet need that motivates behavior at that level (Figure 2.3).

The domination of physical needs drives behavior at the power moral level. At this level "might makes right"; we do something because we want to, we can, and no one can stop us. Our actions are controlled only by someone with greater physical or material power who can provide punishments and rewards. The domination of safety and security needs drives behavior at the deals moral level. At this level we still take what we want if we can, but with those who have more power we make self-serving bargains and compromises in order to get what we want or avoid what we don't want. The domination of the need for love drives behavior at the good boy/good girl moral level. At this level we do what someone else wants in order to be a "good boy" or a "good girl" and win their acceptance, approval, and love. The domination of belonging needs drives behavior at the rules or authority moral level. At this level we follow the rules of the group so that its members will accept and approve of us and we will belong. Identity is solidified in conjunction with the group and the rules become such an integral part of who we are that they guide long after we have moved away from the particular group. The domination of esteem needs drives behavior at the social contracts moral level. At this level we work for the general welfare, for the most good for the most people, not for personal interest. This is the level of the U.S. Constitution. The domination of self-actualization needs drives behavior at the individual conscience moral level. At this level we are guided and motivated by the worth of each individual and by principles of life such as dignity, justice, responsibility, freedom, and equality.

FIGURE 2.3

Maslow's Hierarchy of Needs Correlated with Kohlberg's Moral Levels.

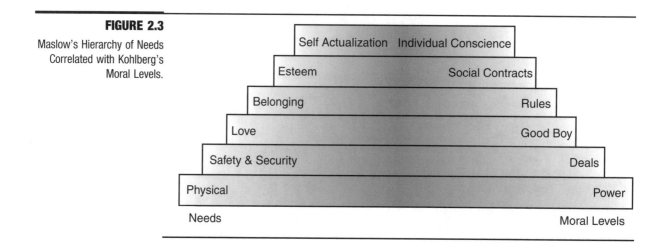

Self Actualization   Individual Conscience

Esteem   Social Contracts

Belonging   Rules

Love   Good Boy

Safety & Security   Deals

Physical   Power

Needs   Moral Levels

EMOTIONAL DEVELOPMENT

The goal of childhood is to allow time to experience and interact with the environment in order to develop strategies (feelings, beliefs, thoughts, emotions, and actions) to meet needs one level at a time until at adulthood we are capable of meeting all of our needs. The feelings we learn to use are the subject of what Erik Erikson called emotional development. Unconscious areas of the brain identify a lack of something that we require. This lack is communicated to the conscious mind by way of neurotransmitters that produce feelings. But not everyone feels the same in the same situation. Based on their feelings in a room full of strangers, some confidently introduce themselves and strike up a conversation while others find an out-of-the-way table and sit alone. Some part of this is surely genetic, but much of it is determined by our emotional development as we respond to the world of our childhood. Erik Erikson (1963, 1982) described this **emotional development** as a set of eight dilemmas that must be resolved as we grow. The way we resolve these determines our feelings, which create the foundation for our emotions and actions.

Trust versus Mistrust

For about the first one to two years of life the child is developing neurons that create the ability to feel trust and/or mistrust. Movement through this or any other stage is the result of physical development of the brain, so the exact timing varies somewhat from child to child. Passage to a new level is more like flowing through increasingly lighter shades of gray rather than abruptly stepping from black to white. The degree of trust or mistrust a person develops has far-ranging effects. The child who is well and lovingly cared for—whose parents are trustworthy—learns that the world is essentially a good place and that the overwhelming power the world possesses is at work for their welfare. The ability to trust also allows them to hope, to have faith, not just in the world, but in themselves. Children see themselves as the center of the universe, so if they learn to trust the world, at the same time and in the same way they learn to trust themselves. If they are harshly treated, neglected, or abused, they learn to mistrust the world and themselves. As groups of neurons develop and lock-in the ability to feel trust or mistrust the foundation for a life is laid, and a life built on trust is very different from a life built on mistrust.

Autonomy versus Doubt

From about 18 months to 3 ½ years children move through the next stage of development. Those who learn to trust the world and themselves have a decided advantage as they attempt to develop a sense of autonomy—the freedom to be themselves, to confidently act on their feelings. A 3-month-old baby is able to see and be very interested in an object, but if the object is removed from sight, it is removed from existence. The baby cannot hold the object in its mind as an image. This complex ability develops quickly, however, and by the age of two it is well developed. The toddler now can create and hold mental images of the multitude of intriguing objects in his or her world. These mental images are symbols that represent the physical object, but they are incomplete. The child has no idea of what the objects feel, taste, or sound like. What happens if you put it in milk? Turn it over? Can it be thrown? Carried? Sat on? The tremendous information base compiled in this stage is utilized throughout life.

The explorations of the child need to be encouraged but structured. A tremendous curiosity drives feelings that take the child out to discover the world. But if the child's reaching out in wonder leads to frequently slapped hands and harsh words, the child quickly comes to doubt the feelings and him or herself. Likewise if children are given no structure, they will walk up to vicious dogs, stick their fingers in electric sockets, touch hot objects, climb up and fall off things. Again the burning curiosity inside is getting them hurt, and they come to doubt themselves and the world. A child in this stage needs structure that insures safety and the permission to be free within that structure.

Initiative versus Guilt

The child who develops trust in the world becomes autonomous and explores, the child who mistrusts comes to doubt and feel shame. From about 3 ½ to 5 years of age trust and autonomy become Initiative, a feeling that leads to action. Mistrust and Doubt become Guilt, the tendency to respond to needs with shame and avoidance. Taking action allows the child to learn how to get needs met. Shame and avoidance set the child up not to act or to act in ways that are not effective in meeting needs.

Mastery versus Inferiority

The next step begins with entry into formal education at about 5 years of age and extends to about 13 years. The child who trusts becomes autonomous and takes initiative. This leads to needs being met and a tremendous amount of learning. The continuation of this process leads to a feelings of mastery and confidence. Children see themselves as being capable of making and doing things; meeting, making, and keeping friends; negotiating with the world and getting what they need. Their direct behaviors are easily modified and they learn and are successful at doing the things necessary to find affection and acceptance. Mistrust leads to Doubt and Guilt. Mistrusting children shrink back inside themselves and develop a sense of Inferiority. They have little belief in their ability to negotiate with the world to successfully get needs met. They most often do not feel loved or accepted and may become angry with the world, but inside they are convinced that they do not deserve the love, care, attention, friendship, possessions, and so on that other people do.

Identity versus Role Confusion

From about 13 to 20 years of age adolescents either establish their Identity or move into Role Confusion. After some experimentation with roles adolescents with a sense of mastery establish their identity. They know themselves and their capabilities. They assume that the world will accept them and they approach it with confidence. Most often the world does accept them and they continue their positive relationship with it. Children who mistrust the world and themselves, who doubt their feelings and feel guilty about needing, and who develop a sense of inferiority are not in a position to simply "be themselves." The deep, unspoken, often even unrecognized, assumption is that, "if others really know me, they won't like me." These adolescents begin to put on any identity that the person or group they are with at the moment will accept. They begin to play roles. And since the role has nothing to do with who they really are, it can be easily changed to fit different groups or people. These teenagers may develop multiple well-defined roles across many different groups. Some of these roles may be very successful and the adolescent may at last win acceptance. But they are painfully aware that it isn't really them who is being accepted, rather it is the role they are playing.

Intimacy versus Isolation

Eventually the young adult develops a more intense relationship with someone in particular and moves either toward Intimacy or Isolation. Those who have followed the line of trust and have developed a clear identity are free to be themselves and have no trouble letting a partner know who they really are—what they like and don't like, when they are angry, happy, sad, excited. Their trust creates the expectation that they will be understood and accepted and gives them the freedom to take risks, to become vulnerable. They let their partner inside and the relationship becomes not only intense, but intimate.

Those who have moved from mistrust through role diffusion eventually play a role well enough to develop an intense relationship. However, they are not free to be themselves. Feelings of doubt, guilt, and inferiority cause them to believe that if their partner really knows them, he or she won't want them. So they keep their partner outside and continue to pretend to be someone they are not. They can be married for 40 years and their partner will never really know them; they build a wall and are isolated behind it.

Generativity versus Self-Absorption

Adults who are intimate are able to let their partner know what they need and behave in ways that motivate the partner to fulfill those needs. The needs, having been met, do not dominate feelings and actions. When we are not dominated by our own needs and feelings we are able to see things as others see them and consider what others, especially children, need for healthy emotional development. We are able to be nurturing and supportive. In addition, the immature behavior of others does not threaten us and we are able to focus on finding solutions to problems rather than attacking the people who present the problems. This state of positive contribution to the human experience is called generativity.

When we are isolated our partner cannot know what we need and our actions most often move them away from doing things that would meet those needs. As with hunger or thirst, any need that is chronically unmet grows increasingly stronger until it becomes the focus of existence. Resentment builds. It is common to hear those in this position talk bitterly about doing everything for everyone else while no one does anything for them. They have so thoroughly hidden themselves in the roles they are playing that no one really knows them, or how to meet their needs. In this state we are not free to see things as others see them, but color everything with how it meets or can be made to meet our own needs. This self-absorption does not leave us in any position to understand what others think, feel, or need and our unproductive, self-serving behaviors cannot meet the needs of others, not even those of our own children.

Dignity versus Despair

As we age we begin to lose. We may lose physical appearance and abilities, mental acuity, eyesight, hearing, our profession, loved ones, our home. We may go to live in a nursing home where we can lose the right to decide when and what we eat, when we go to bed and get up, when and what medicine we take, when we see our children. Some of us will be the little old gentleman or lady who sits alone in a wheelchair for hours at a time in the nursing home hallway, urgently clinging to anyone who will talk to us.

The degree of loss will differ, but we will all lose part of ourselves, our lives, our loves. Those who have been fortunate enough to trust and learn to deal effectively with the world will enter this time of life from the phase of generativity. They will be happy and satisfied with their lives and who they are, have self-respect, and above all else, integrity and dignity. All else can be taken away, but nothing can touch these. These older adults are easy to see in any nursing home. They are the ones who take an active interest in what is going on, in their neighbors, the staff, in activities. They make life more pleasant for those around them, and are especially appreciated by the staff.

Those who are living self-absorbed, unfulfilled lives when they enter this time of life will not be so lucky. They will see life as a series of missed opportunities and failed relationships. They will be bitter with a world that has never cared for them or met their needs. Their physical losses will be seen as the final betrayal and they will despair. It is also easy to identify them in any nursing home. They seem to be angry most of the time and are not as invested in the activities or with the people in the home. They often strike out verbally and physically, inflicting what they feel inside onto those around them, especially the staff.

PERSONALITY TRAITS

As we learn from experience and develop the emotions and actions we need to get our needs met, our genetic tendencies are molded and shaped into specific **personality traits**. Robert McCrae and Paul Costa have identified five such traits that can be measured to describe personality (Wiggins & Trapnell, 1997; John & Srivastava, 1999).

Extraversion

This trait describes a person's engagement with the world. People who score high in **extraversion** are emotionally positive and energetic; they tend to be upbeat, friendly, outgoing, sociable, and assertive and they like attention. Those who score low lack this energy and activity level. They tend to be quiet, low-key, deliberate, and independent, preferring to be alone.

Agreeableness

Agreeableness describes a person's concern with social harmony and cooperation. Agreeable people tend to be cooperative, sympathetic, trusting, modest, and straightforward. Disagreeable people tend to be more concerned with self-interest than in getting along with others and can be suspicious, uncooperative, and unfriendly.

Conscientiousness

This trait reflects the way we control our impulses. **Conscientious** people tend to be disciplined and well organized, diligent, punctual, and dependable. Impulsive people can be seen by others as colorful and fun to be with, but impulsiveness places more importance on immediate rather than delayed gratification and can be destructive to a person's personal, social, and professional relationships.

Neuroticism

Neuroticism describes a person's tendency to have negative feelings. People who are emotionally negative tend to be anxious, hostile, insecure, vulnerable, and self-conscious. People who score low in neuroticism tend to be emotionally stable, secure, and calm.

Openness to Experience

This trait distinguishes conventional from unconventional thinking. People with **openness to experience** tend to be curious, imaginative, flexible, individualistic, non-conforming, and often artistic. Closed thinking is conservative and resists change, preferring the familiar and regarding the arts and sciences as having little practical value.

SUMMARY

Our DNA provides the plans for our personality traits and if everything is OK, we will grow according to that plan. But everything may not be OK. Everyone has the same set of needs. Their environment will either meet these needs or not; if it does not their development will be affected. Psychological functioning is affected in the same way. We become dominated by the lowest need we cannot learn to meet. That chronically unmet need will grow powerful and motivate behaviors generally typical to the corresponding moral level. As we move through the stages of emotional development we establish groups of neurons with thousands of connections capable of recreating the emotions we have learned. We may have the DNA to be extraverted emotionally positive and energetic, upbeat, friendly, outgoing, sociable, and assertive. The expression of that trait can be strengthened by an environment that leads us to trust, act on our feelings, and take initiative; or weakened by an environment that leads us to mistrust, doubt our feelings, and feel guilty about the things we want. We will have a genetic tendency to score high or low on each of the personality traits. This is the beginning point. Where we ultimately wind up is determined by how these genetic predispositions are molded by the world we grow in. Personality traits represent the sum of the feelings we have learned to respond with, the beliefs we use to appraise these feelings, the emotions the feelings become, and the actions the emotions drive. These tend to be strongly self-perpetuating because they have as their foundation the physical structure of the brain.

APPLICATION SKILL

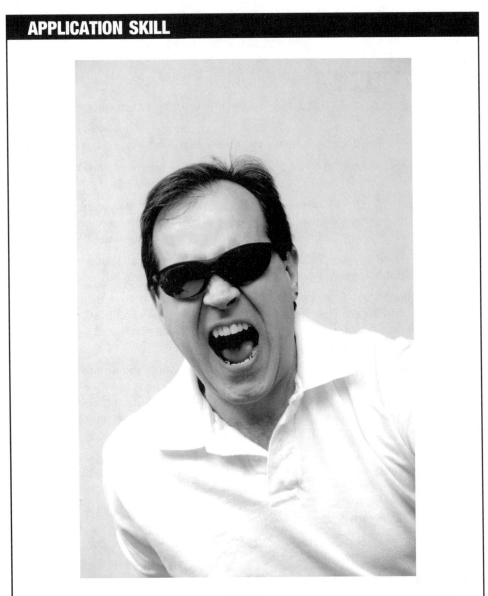

Wait

Using the skill of really looking at the client, what is your reaction to the person you see in this photograph? If you had to deal with him how do you think you would approach him? What do you think you would feel?

APPLICATION SKILL *(continued)*

In making appraisals of others, we tend to spend no more time or effort than necessary for a quick decision (Operario & Fiske, 2001). This efficiency saves time and effort at the risk of being inaccurate. Look a little longer, a little deeper. The purpose of looking is to see, to understand, not to simply react.

Act, do not react.

Our brain is forever searching for patterns and for ways to organize and interpret information, but we are far from infallible—we even see animals and faces in the clouds. Just as we realize that the animal is not really in the cloud we need to come to realize that our appraisal of someone is not really that person.

Avoiding hasty and negative judgments can hinge on the simple things we say to ourselves in the first moments. Rather than saying impatient, critical, or judgmental things to ourselves about the client we should be asking ourselves; "who is this person in front of me?"; "what makes this behavior necessary?"; and "how can I help?"

CONCEPT REVIEW

personality – A set of traits that stays the same over time and from one situation to the next.

genetic plans – In the DNA present the model for each trait.

environment – Determines how the genetic plan will be expressed and the final form of the trait.

cognitive stages – The brain moves through four stages of development, focused on specific developmental tasks in order to give a child the time to experience the world and master simple tasks first before moving on to more complex ones.

sensorimotor – 0 to 2 years. Feelings created by sensory input (hunger, cold, etc.) lead directly to motor (physical) responses with little complex processing.

symbolic functions – 2 to 7 years. The ability to create and maintain mental images and symbols and to express them as language develops rapidly. Children learn and use self-advancing bargains and compromises to stay safe and secure and to get what they want or avoid what they don't want.

concrete functions – 7 to 11 years. Logic and reason develop and are used in a black or white manner, dealing with what is present in the moment in order to gain what is wanted or avoid what is not wanted. Approval, affection, and acceptance are sought from those holding power in the family, and in the group. Sexuality develops.

formal operations – 12+ years. Higher mental functions requiring abstract thought emerge. The ability to understand and use principles, think through alternatives, and base behavior on beliefs of what should be develops. Needs for recognition and respect from others grow into the need for self-respect, requiring motivation and direction from within.

psychological model – A theoretical construct used to describe, explain, and predict psychological functioning.

proposed psychological model – The model proposed begins with the unconscious part of the brain detecting a lack of some element necessary for individuals to survive, develop friendships and associations, mate, protect and nurture their young, or to be fully themselves. This lack is a need and it is communicated to the conscious part of the brain by way of neurotransmitters that create a feeling. The individual processes this feeling along with other information such as the who, what, when, and where of the situation, established beliefs about self and others, and probable outcomes of various actions. These are encapsulated into self-talk, which changes the feeling into an emotion. The emotion powers an action. Together the emotion and action comprise a behavior. The goal of the behavior is to supply the element necessary to relieve the original lack and meet the need, enabling the individual to survive, develop friendships and associations, mate, protect and nurture their young, or to be true to their own nature.

Maslow's hierarchy of needs – Abraham Maslow proposed that needs exist in an order from lowest to highest, and that lower needs must be fulfilled before higher needs can emerge. These needs are physical, safety and security, love and belonging, esteem, and self-actualization. The lowest need that is not adequately fulfilled will grow to dominate as neurotransmitters are produced, creating feelings that drive the person toward fulfilling the need.

Kohlberg's moral levels – Maslow's hierarchy establishes multiple levels of needs that must be met in order. Over time the lowest level need that is consistently unmet grows ever more powerful until it motivates thoughts, emotions, and actions at that level. This motivation is the key to moral levels. Moral levels are defined not by what we do, but by why we do it. As the lowest order need that is chronically unmet grows powerful it motivates behavior that can often be described by the characteristics of the moral at that level.

Erikson's emotional dilemmas – Erik Erikson proposed a set of eight emotional dilemmas that each person must resolve as part of the development process. These dilemmas exist as a set of extremes, and the individual will become established at some point on a continuum between the two. The point at which a person becomes established is determined by genetic predisposition and interactions with the environment. Erikson's dilemmas are trust versus mistrust; autonomy versus doubt and shame; initiative versus guilt; industry versus inferiority; identity versus role confusion; intimacy versus isolation; generativity versus self absorption; and integrity versus despair.

five trait personality theory – Robert McCrae and Paul Costa have identified five traits that can be measured to describe personality. These traits represent an extreme of personality and each has an opposite. The trait a person develops will establish itself somewhere along the continuum between the two extremes. The point on the continuum at which a trait becomes established is determined by genetic predisposition and interactions with the environment. These five personality traits are extraversion, agreeableness, conscientiousness, neuroticism, and openness to experience.

the five personality traits and their opposites – Extraversion and introversion; neuroticism and emotional stability; openness to experience and closed thinking; agreeableness and disagreeableness; and conscientiousness and impulsiveness.

personality development – Our DNA provides plans for each personality trait. How thoroughly the genetic plan is implemented depends on interactions with the environment. The final personality trait is influenced both by heredity and by the environment. Once established, personality traits strongly tend to be enduring because they are locked into the physical structure of the brain.

REVIEW QUESTIONS

I.   Completion

Complete the following sentences.

1. Jean Piaget described a series of four _____ from infancy to adulthood.

2. The highest order need in Maslow's hierarchy is _____.

3. Erik Erikson described emotional development as a set of eight _____ we must resolve as we grow.

4. Autonomy is the freedom to _____.

5. Neuroticism describes a person's tendency to have _____ feelings.

II.   Multiple Choice

Select the letter of the choice that best completes the statement.

6. Personality can best be described as a set of
   A. Drives
   B. Genetic predispositions
   C. Learned tendencies
   D. Stable characteristics

7. The stage of cognitive development in which physical sensations lead directly to motor responses is
   A. Sensorimotor
   B. Symbolic functions
   C. Concrete functions
   D. Formal operations

8. The stage of cognitive development in which logic and reason develop and are used in a black or white manner is
   A. Sensorimotor
   B. Symbolic functions
   C. Concrete functions
   D. Formal operations

9. In the psychological model the purpose of an action is
   A. To respond to other people
   B. To get needs met
   C. To influence other people
   D. To respond to feelings

10. In the psychological model, self-talk reflects:
    A. Our appraisal of the situation
    B. What we think we should do
    C. Our understanding of what is being said
    D. Our opinion of the person we are speaking with

III.   Matching

Match each term with its correct description.

   A. Dislike change
   B. Trust
   C. Behaviors
   D. Enduring
   E. Formal operations

Emotions and actions together are _____

The cognitive stage that enables us to think in the abstract terms needed to feel empathy for another is _____

Closed thinking: _____

To remain consistent over time and from one situation to the next is _____

Autonomy is built on _____

IV.   Critical Thinking

11. What is the advantage and disadvantage of personality traits that are enduring?

12. On the five trait personality inventory, if a person scored low on extraversion, low on neuroticism, high on openness to experience, high on agreeableness, and moderate on conscientiousness, how would you expect them to act in a social setting with a group of strangers?

13. How might the motivation for behavior described by moral levels relate to unmet needs?

14. In a position that required independently traveling to many locations and assertively dealing with new people, what combination of personality traits do you think would offer the most advantage? Why?

15. Why do needs that are chronically unfulfilled grow to dominate behavior?

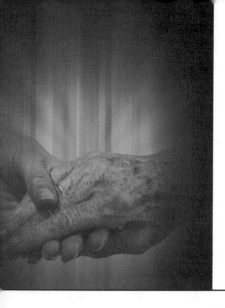

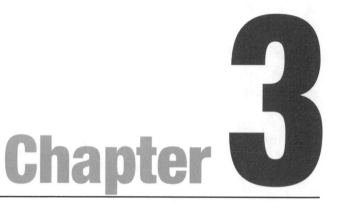

Chapter 3

Upon completion of this chapter you should be able to:

1. Give an example of how the environment can limit the expression of genetic plans.
2. Describe individualistic and collectivist cultures.
3. Describe the effect of the community and status within the community on the child.
4. List and define six parenting styles.
5. Describe the probable effect on adult behavior of being raised in each of the six parenting styles listed.
6. Describe the law of probability and relate it to the probable affects of parenting styles.

KEY TERMS

environment	parenting style	conditional parenting
culture	neglect	assertive parenting
individualistic culture	passive aggression	supportive parenting
collectivistic culture	active aggression	probability
status	coercion	
parent	indulgence	

The Environment

APPLICATION SKILL

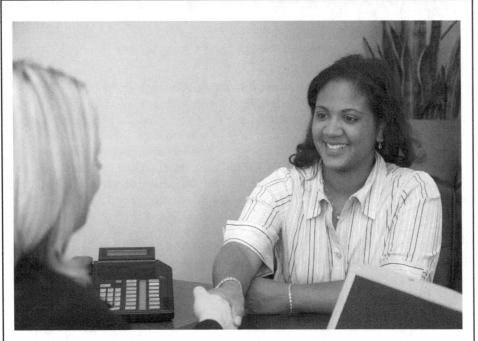

Listen

You have really looked at the person in front of you. You have waited to form an impression of them. Now it is time to listen.

Scenario

An elderly female patient has been recently admitted to the nursing facility where you are employed. Her adult children have visited regularly since her arrival. The daughter with whom the patient had lived, and who had cared for her prior to her admission, expresses sadness at her inability to meet her mother's needs but is friendly and appreciative of the good care provided. But the daughter who did not provide direct care for her mother prior to admission is often angry and hostile, continuously finding fault with even the smallest issues regarding her mother's care. How do you understand and respond to the sadness of the first daughter, and the rude, hostile, at times angry overreactions of the second?

INTRODUCTION

This chapter is about the environment that children grow up in. It is consistent interactions with the environment that stimulate the development of neurons and determine the expression of genetic predispositions that create personality. Many things come together to create an environment. The culture provides the setting the community exists within. The community provides the setting the family exists within, with the family occupying a very specific status within that community. The family provides the setting the child exists within. Of all the factors that affect the child, the most influential is the parenting style. All of these factors combined create a strong probability for how the child will react, but they do not create the child's destiny.

Look for the basic cultural types and the effect of status in the community on the family and the child. Also look for six parenting styles, the probable effect of each of these on the child, and the reason that you can never be completely sure of how any one specific child will respond to any of these.

After reading this chapter you should have a clearer understanding of how the environment can modify the expression of genetic plans, be able to define two cultural types, explain the affect of status, describe six specific parenting styles and their probable affects on the child, and understand why some children seem to defy all of the odds.

THE ENVIRONMENT

The growth of the brain and the development of personality begin with a set of genetic plans; but plans are only intentions. The final outcome depends on how the expression of those plans is modified by interactions with the environment. A person may have the genetic plan to be six feet tall, but if he or she is malnourished and has poor health care he or she may only grow to five-and-a-half feet. The **environment** is the immediate world that surrounds a child. Culture, people, location, buildings, schools, automobiles, economy, animals, and status are elements of the environment that have an affect on the development of the child. The first element of the environment is the culture.

Culture

Most regional cultures exist on a spectrum somewhere between the extremes of two basic cultural types. An **Individualistic culture** values independence and personal responsibility. Individuals are given a great degree of autonomy and freedom but are seen as being responsible for obeying basic rules of ethics and law and for meeting their own needs. There is little safety net, with only very basic needs provided for should a person not be capable of providing for themselves. At the opposite extreme a **collectivistic culture** values conformity to group values and rules and there is considerable pressure on individuals to conform to shared beliefs and behaviors. There is usually a large safety net and a wide range of needs are provided for should a person not be capable of providing for themselves. The community exists within the culture. Religion is usually an expression of the culture. Eastern Confucianism teaches respect for traditional values, beliefs, and practices and is purely collectivistic. The Moslem religion, eastern religion and philosophy in general, and some western religions such as the Amish and Mormons tend toward collectivism. Western philosophy in general tends toward individualism. The basic philosophies and beliefs of individuals within a community and what is required to achieve high status within that community are for the most part determined by the culture.

Status

Status is created by the territory that we establish within the community (see Chapter 1 for a more complete discussion of status and territory). High-status families within a culture most often attend better schools and are treated better in general than are low-status families. The personality traits we develop guide us in the choices we make, but what we have to choose from is provided by the family and the community we live in and by our family's position within that community. The subculture of poverty, with its substandard schools, low expectations, and lack of encouragement and opportunity tends to be self-perpetuating, as does the subculture of privilege, no matter what larger culture they are a part of. We are molded by our environment and, once formed, personality traits are enduring. For the most part we simply adapt to the culture and position we are raised in, accepting the family structure, parenting beliefs, religion, value system, and vocational choices that culture and position provides.

Parenting Style

The culture, the community, and the family's relative status within the community all have a profound effect on the development of the child, but none is as powerful as the parent. The **parent** is the person or people who provide primary care for the child. A person may become a parent by biology, marriage, foster care, adoption, or just by being there. None of these guarantees that the person will be a parent to a child, and none excludes the possibility. In the end, for good or ill, the child's parent, the one who has the greatest influence on development, is the one who most regularly interacts with and cares for the child. There are many ways to parent a child and each approach requires something different from the child. We are all human and all have the same basic needs. Our genetic code tells us what we need and gives us the starting points for each trait of our personality; but our parents allow or do not allow that personality to be expressed, and teach us how we can, and even *if* we can, get our needs met. There is a lot of difference in parenting styles, and even in how one person parents at different times. No one is anything all of the time. Very gentle parents can sometimes be harsh, and very harsh parents can be gentle. Remember that in the development of the brain it is consistency that counts. Neurons and pathways that are used a lot grow strong and efficient; those used little do not. Unless they are complicated by deeply felt, enduring emotions such as the perception of being loved greatly or of being betrayed, or by a required change such as having to keep a dark secret, a few experiences out of the ordinary will not greatly affect a child. Far more important are the consistent experiences children have every day. Each parent has a **parenting style** created by their personality characteristics, their history, their current situation, and their beliefs. While no two parents are exactly alike, there are some patterns, some general parenting styles.

Parenting Styles Defined

Neglect is the consistent tendency to ignore the child. In this situation the child's physical needs are not taken care of, but more than that the child is not given the ability to interact with the world. Remember that interaction with the environment, which for a baby and young child is the parent, generates the growth and development of the brain, and that neurons that are not used die and go away forever. Neglected children have a much smaller, less-developed brain than non-neglected children, and if the neglect is severe enough, they lose forever the potential to live anything like a normal life. For this reason neglected babies often give up, go into failure to thrive, and die. As adults, neglected children often live withdrawn, hopeless lives, constantly snatching defeat out of the jaws of victory. They very often neglect their own children, passing the legacy down from generation to generation to generation. At times they may use **passive aggression**, attempting to sabotage or harm others by indirect means so as to not take responsibility for their actions. **Active aggression**, that is, direct violence, is less likely, but may be explosive when it happens.

Coercion is the use of force or the realistic threat of force to get children to do what the parent wants. It is always accompanied by either physical or emotional abuse, because threats alone lose their power in time if the child is not either hurt occasionally or hurt severely enough initially to leave a permanent impression. Coercive parents get their children to do what they want by yelling, threatening, and punishing. Children are told to obey "because I said so," and when offered, explanations tend to be accusations. The parent is reacting out of his or her own unmet needs and insecurities, not out of concern for the best interest of the child, and when the baby grows into a toddler he or she runs into a barrage of anger and slaps, which continue in slightly different forms throughout childhood. As with neglect, there are many degrees of coercion. If treated severely enough a coerced child may react much like a neglected child and withdraw, afraid to try, afraid to even be seen. More often the coerced child becomes oppositional, even defiant, and may be passively or actively aggressive.

Indulgence gives children no limits. Their parents either allow them to do as they please or make only feeble attempts at control, giving in whenever the child pleads or has tantrums. In addition, the parent most often protects the child when they get into trouble in the community, refusing to allow them to experience the consequences of their own behavior. Indulged children soon develop a sense of entitlement, believing that the world should give them what they want and that life should be easy. But as the child grows older the parent cannot control the world for them, and when the parent fails at making life easy the indulged person, who has developed very few coping skills, is hurt and betrayed, and may live the rest of their life angry and resentful at a world that refuses to give them what their parents did, and at parents who have failed in their self-imposed promise to make life easy.

Conditional parenting means, "I like you and I love you if you do what I want, but I do not like you and I do not love you if you do not." Where coercion uses physical or emotional pain to force compliance, conditional parenting uses rejection. No matter how hard a child tries he or she can never please the parent all the time, and the inevitable rejection soon teaches that the child is worth nothing: it is only what they are seen to do that matters. This may lead to a desperate effort to comply with authority that can last a lifetime; it may lead to continual manipulations; or it may lead to resentment and opposition. The ultimate in conditional parenting was the "tough love" movement of the 1980s that responded to adolescent resentment and disobedience by throwing a host of fourteen- to sixteen-year-old children out of their homes and into the streets where they were forced to prostitute themselves to survive. The claim of the movement was that love for the child motivated the rejection, but the will of the parent, not the good of the child, was the primary consideration.

Assertive parenting is making and consistently enforcing rules in the best interests of the child. Decisions are made not for the convenience or due to the mood of the parent, but genuinely because the parent wants what is best for the child. The child is not included in making the rules because the parent is in a much better position to know what the child needs. Once a decision is made it is consistently enforced, but love is never withheld and the child is never made to feel rejected. It is made clear that the behavior, not the child, is the issue. Children of assertive parents soon learn that it is best to cooperate with a world that is genuinely trying to help them and they generally succeed well in school and on the job. What they do not learn is how to question authority or how to resolve issues if they disagree with authority. As adults, rather than openly disagree they tend to harbor resentments and eventually leave a situation rather than work to change it.

Supportive parenting has much in common with assertive parenting. Rules are made and consistently enforced in the best interests of the child, but with supportive parenting the child is always included in making the rules and can always question a decision after it is made, provided that the questioning is done in an appropriate manner. An appropriate manner means that the child thinks through what they believe is wrong with the rule and how they think it should be changed. If the child's position makes sense, even from a child's perspective, the rule is modified, as long as the change does not harm the child. If the rule is not changed the parent carefully explains to the child how they believe the change would be bad for the child or otherwise is not possible. The parent makes the final decision. If the rule is changed the new rule is consistently enforced; if it is not changed the original rule remains and is consistently enforced. The child of a supportive parent also quickly learns that it is best to cooperate with a world that is working for their good. But unlike the child of an assertive parent, they learn that if they disagree they have the right to express that disagreement, as long as they do it in a logical, productive manner. As adults they are more prone to talk about and try to resolve problems, and more likely to work through issues rather than harbor resentments or leave.

PROBABILITY

Each parenting style and culture represents a consistent pattern of interactions with the child that combine with the child's unique genetic predispositions, resulting in the development of the brain and the emerging personality. But there is a wild card in the deck. You can never overlook the effects of pure chance. Everything in the universe, including how a child will respond to a specific parenting style, school environment, or culture, is subject to the law of **probability**. That is because everything in the universe is created from quantum waves, which are waves of pure probability; and everything has that probability imbedded into the very fabric of its being. To explain probability I'll use the example of human intelligence (Figure 3.1).

The average IQ is 100. The normal intelligence range is one standard step (deviation) above or below the average—between 85 and 115. Sixty-six and two-thirds percent of people have an IQ within the normal range. Fourteen and two-thirds percent have an IQ in the range of two standard steps above—115 to 130—and two standard steps below—70 to 85—the average. Two percent have an IQ greater than two standard steps above—higher than 130—and two standard steps below—less than 70—the average.

This is the standard probability curve, and it isn't just a rule of science, it is a law of science. Because of it, gambling isn't a gamble for the casino house. All the house has to do is set the odds in its favor by a few percentage points and attract enough people to keep the dollar volume high. The odds will deliver like clockwork. Probability describes everything. How intelligent will babies be? How fast can horses run? How tall will trees grow? How will people respond to a medical treatment? Smoking two packs of cigarettes a day, what are my chances of contracting lung cancer? Never having smoked in my life, what are my chances of contracting lung cancer? It also describes the probability of how children will respond to a particular parenting style. Sixty-seven percent of children will respond in a normal way to a particular parenting style. Fourteen and two-thirds percent will respond better than you would have expected and fourteen and two-thirds percent will respond worse than you would have expected. Two percent will respond remarkably well, and two percent will respond remarkably poorly. Just as there are people who smoke all of their lives and never have lung cancer, there are those who are raised in severe dysfunction but are normal and happy. And just as there are people who never smoke yet who have lung cancer, there are those who are raised in normal, healthy environments but are dysfunctional. Not smoking does not guarantee that you will not have lung cancer, it just lowers the probability; and smoking doesn't guarantee lung cancer, it just raises the probability. Growing up in a healthy home environment doesn't guarantee an emotionally healthy adult, but it does raise the probability dramatically, and growing up in a

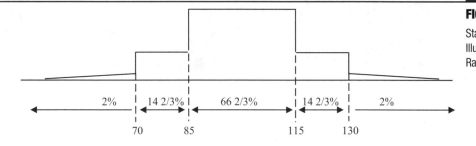

FIGURE 3.1

Standard Probability Curve Illustrating the Normal IQ Range.

dysfunctional family does not guarantee that you will be dysfunctional, but it does also dramatically increase the probability. Probability is flawless at predicting the outcome when dealing with large numbers, but it is useless at determining the outcome of one specific case. It does reveal the odds of a particular response, but one individual may emerge in the two-thirds normal population or appear in the two percent at either end. There is no way to predict the outcome of individual development.

SUMMARY

The development of the brain ultimately results in personality traits. These traits begin with our DNA, but where they and the beliefs, emotions, and actions we learn to express them with end up is decided by the environment. The environment that influences the growth of children is complex. The culture provides the setting in which the community exists. The community provides the setting in which the family exists. The family's status establishes the family's position within the community. The family provides the setting in which the parent(s) exist. And the parent(s) provide the setting in which the child exists. Each level has a deep influence. The community and the family's position in the community have a powerful affect on the beliefs, practices, and values of the family and on the child, but the most powerful aspect of a child's environment is the parent. This chapter lists six parenting styles from very negative, with very negative consequences for the child, to very positive, with very positive consequences for the child. But how one specific child will respond to a specific community and parenting style cannot be predicted. Most children will respond negatively to a negative parenting style and positively to a positive parenting style, but some children will respond better, and a few much better than you would expect, and some will respond worse, and a few much worse than you would expect.

APPLICATION SKILL

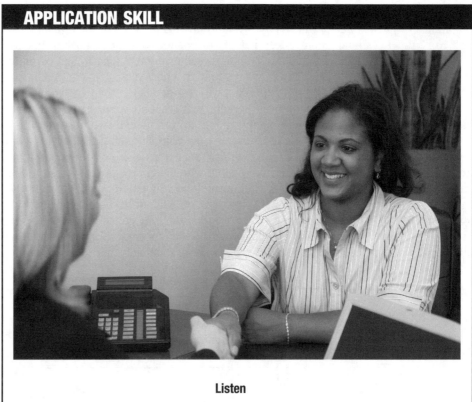

Listen

You have really looked at the person in front of you. You have waited to form an impression of them. Now it is time to listen.

APPLICATION SKILL *(continued)*

Active Listening

The loss of health, whether from injury, disease, or years, often brings with it grief and distress. That distress can deeply affect the emotions of patients and their families. It may collapse inward into sadness and depression or it can erupt outward as dissatisfaction and anger. It is important to remember that your patient's well-being is directly tied to the well-being of their family and respond in a supportive way to the emotions of both. The most supportive response you can make is to actively listen. To actively pursue something is to purposely act to bring it about. To be passive is to sit back and wait to see if it will come to you. Active listening is purposely engaging the person in conversation and focusing on the process of listening to ensure that you have really heard what they are saying. It is you taking responsibility for understanding rather than making the other person responsible for explaining. To do that you have to really see the person in front of you, focus on them; do not allow yourself to be distracted by other things going on around you, or by anything about them—what they are wearing, how they are speaking, or how they look. Give them your full attention and let them know they have it. Look them in the eye (try to get at eye level); unfold your arms; do not fidget; listen to what they are saying. Do not judge what they are saying, do not think about how to reply, focus everything on making sure that you hear and understand. Encourage them to express themselves and ensure that you have all of the information by using short, appropriate statements or questions like "you feel strongly about this," or by rephrasing their statements: "Are you saying that …?" Practice this. You will find people opening up and talking to you in ways that you may have never experienced; and as they express themselves the emotion inside finds a release, and the reason for the sadness or anger diminishes. You do not need to make promises or try to resolve their issues; really listening to people is one of the most supporting, accepting, and respecting things you can do, and even if you are with them for only a few minutes, people do respond.

CONCEPT REVIEW

the environment – The immediate world that surrounds a child. People, location, buildings, schools, automobiles, economy, animals, culture, and status are all elements of the environment and all have an effect on the development of the child.

culture – The values, traditions, and belief system of a community of people.

individualistic culture – A culture that values independence and personal responsibility. Individuals are given a great degree of autonomy and freedom but are seen as being responsible for obeying basic rules of ethics and law and for meeting their own needs.

collectivistic culture – A culture that values conformity to group values and rules. There is considerable pressure on individuals to conform to shared beliefs and behaviors.

community – The setting (culture, location, occupation, people) in which the family exists.

status – The family's relative position within the community.

parent(s) – The person or people who provide primary care for the child. A person may become a parent by biology, marriage, foster care, adoption, or just by being there.

parenting style – A consistent pattern of interactions between a parent and a child created by the personality characteristics, history, and beliefs of the parent and by the current situation.

neglect – A parenting style in which the parent has the consistent tendency to ignore the child. The child's physical needs are not taken care of, but more than that the child is not given the ability to interact with the world to generate the growth and development of the brain; neurons that are not used die and go away, forever limiting the child's future potential.

passive aggression – Attempting to harm another either physically or emotionally in such a way as to avoid taking responsibility for the harm inflicted.

active aggression – Direct, open attempts to harm another either physically or emotionally.

coercion – The use of force or the realistic threat of force to get children to do what the parent wants. It is always accompanied by either physical or emotional abuse, because threats alone lose their power in time if the child is not either hurt occasionally or hurt severely enough initially to leave a permanent impression.

indulgence – Giving children no limits. Their parents either allow them to do as they please or make only feeble attempts at control, giving in whenever the child pleads or has tantrums. In addition, the parent most often protects the child when they get into trouble in the community, refusing to allow them to experience the consequences of their own behavior.

conditional parenting – "I like you and I love you if you do what I want, but I do not like you and I do not love you if you do not." No matter how hard a child tries, he or she can never please the parent all the time, and the inevitable rejection soon teaches the child that he or she is worth nothing; it is only what they are seen to do that matters.

assertive parenting – Making and consistently enforcing rules in the best interests of the child. The child is not included in making the rules because the parent believes that they are in a much better position than the child to know what the child needs.

supportive parenting – Also involves making and consistently enforcing rules in the best interests of the child, but with supportive parenting the child is always included in making the rules and can always question a decision after it is made, provided that the questioning is done in an appropriate manner.

probability – A predictable pattern that describes the odds of how one individual will respond to a specific parenting style.

REVIEW QUESTIONS

I.   Completion

Complete the following sentences.

1. Abuse is most often a part of a _____ parenting style.

2. Allowing the child to participate in making and changing rules is part of a _____ parenting style.

3. The parenting style most likely to result in the death of an infant is the _____ parenting style.

4. The parenting style that most severely limits the child's potential is the _____ parenting style.

5. Protecting the child from the consequences of his or her own behavior is part of the _____ parenting style.

II.   Multiple Choice

Select the letter of the choice that best completes the statement.

6. The factor in the environment that has the most affect on brain development is
   A. Love
   B. Discipline
   C. Consistency
   D. Education

7. In conditional parenting the compliance of the child is obtained by using
   A. Rejection
   B. Rules
   C. Consequences
   D. Punishment

8. Passive aggression is
   A. Attempting to harm others indirectly so as to avoid being held accountable for it.
   B. Attempting to harm others by not complying.
   C. Attempting to harm others by any means necessary.
   D. Allowing others to be hurt and doing nothing about it.

9. The percentage of children who will respond in a normal way to a normal environment is
   A. 83.3%
   B. 66.67%
   C. 14.67%
   D. 50%

10. The parenting style that operates for the good of the child but in which the child has no input into rules is
   A. Coercion
   B. Conditional
   C. Supportive
   D. Assertive

III.   Matching

Match each term with its correct description.
   A. Indulgence
   B. Probability
   C. Individualistic
   D. Collectivistic
   E. Parent

_____ An explanation for why some people who smoke all their lives do not contract lung cancer, while others who never smoke do.

_____ The most powerful influence in the development of a child.

_____ A culture that values conformity to group values and practices.

_____ Giving in and allowing a child to have what they want when they have a tantrum.

_____ A culture that values individual freedom and responsibility.

IV.   Critical Thinking

11. What can probabilities predict with certainty about the development of one specific child?

12. Why would an indulged child have trouble coping with life as an adult?

13. How does a family's status in the community affect the way the children are treated by others in the community?

14. How does coercing a child to obtain obedience affect the child's behavior toward others who have less power?

15. Why is the parent the most powerful influence in a child's development?

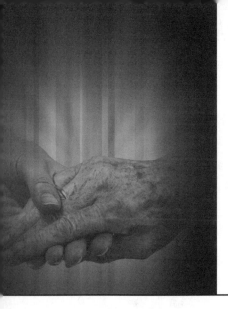

Chapter 4

Upon completion of this chapter you should be able to:

1. Define functional and dysfunctional behavior.
2. Define rational and irrational beliefs.
3. Define adjustment.
4. Define defense mechanism.
5. Describe 14 specific defense mechanisms.
6. Explain the process of change as it applies to human behavior.
7. Explain the role of stress in regression.

KEY TERMS

functional	appraisal	stress
dysfunctional	defense mechanisms	stress reaction
rational	adjustment	
irrational	change	

Function, Dysfunction, and Change

APPLICATION SKILL

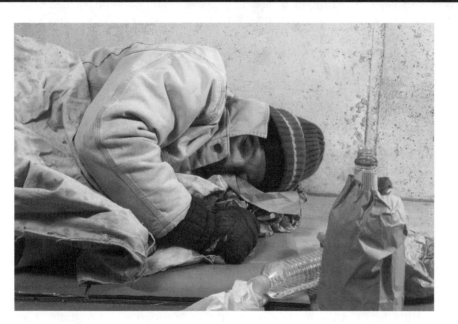

Ask

You have really looked at the person in front of you. You have allowed yourself to feel your response to them but have not judged them. You have listened attentively. Now it is time to ask for the information and understanding that you need.

Scenario

A 40-year-old, drug-addicted resident of the streets is admitted to your hospital with an abscess on his thigh at an injection site. A surgeon performs an incision and drainage and places him on IV antibiotics for 14 days to clear the infection. As the patient withdraws from the drugs he becomes increasingly agitated, angry, rude, and demanding of the staff. On his third day he leaves the hospital, against medical advice (AMA). Nearly two weeks later he returns to the hospital, his thigh significantly worse. The surgeon again performs an incision and drainage and places him on two weeks of IV antibiotics. He again leaves against medical advice after only a few days. On his third admission the infection is severe, possibly into the thigh bone itself. A third incision and drainage is performed and he is again placed on a two-week regimen of IV antibiotics. If he leaves again the overwhelming likelihood is that when he returns his leg will have to be amputated at the hip. The pattern begins to repeat and he becomes increasingly agitated, angry, and rude with the staff as he withdraws from the drugs. It is obvious that he is close to leaving again against medical advice before the infection is cleared. What do you do?

INTRODUCTION

This chapter is about the rapid change that happens in all of our lives and the constant adjustment it takes for us to keep our balance and meet our needs. It is about the irrational beliefs, negative self-talk, and defense mechanisms that can block us from making those adjustments and the dysfunction that can grow if we do not. It is about positive self-talk that can help us and how we can go about changing if we find ourselves in the midst of dysfunction. And finally it is about stress and the hazard it presents to those who have put in the hard work that change requires.

Look for the listings of irrational beliefs, negative and positive self-talk, and defense mechanisms. Pay careful attention to the effect that rapidly mixing cultures has on the ability to adjust, and very careful attention to the process of change and growth and the effect of stress.

After studying this chapter you should have an appreciation for the effect of rapid change, including rapid cultural mixing, on individual adjustment. You should understand the statement "Adjustment is blocked by irrational beliefs, which result in negative self-talk that powers defense mechanisms" and be able to identify some specific examples of irrational beliefs, negative self-talk, and defense mechanisms. In addition, you should have a better insight into the process of change and the hazard of stress.

FUNCTION

Natural genetic tendencies are molded by the environment to produce durable personality traits. We use these traits, and the beliefs and behaviors we have learned to express them with, to interact with others in our environment. If the beliefs and behaviors we have learned are functional, others in our environment will respond to them in such a way as to meet our needs. If they are dysfunctional, they produce a response in others that does not meet our needs. If we want others to not hurt us but to love us, accept us, or respect us we must behave in ways that influence them to do that. It isn't necessary that everyone respond well, but it is necessary that our family, our group, and most people in general do. The factors involved in developing the ability to behave in ways that influence others to meet our needs are amazingly complex. A specific family environment is shaped by the parents as well as by the culture and the family's position within that culture. An individual's beliefs and behaviors are shaped primarily by their family environment. Beliefs and behaviors allow us to interpret the actions of others and respond in appropriate ways. But what is seen as appropriate varies greatly from culture to culture, at multiple status levels within the same culture, and often within separate families at the same level of status in the same culture. This produces wide separations between people. These separations begin with differences in genetic predispositions, but are magnified by the beliefs and behaviors taught by parents, position, and culture. Safety and security come from knowing what to do. If we have no doubt about our ability to meet our physical needs, stay safe and secure, give and receive love, be accepted, and be respected, we are secure and comfortable in our surroundings. We are more comfortable with others who believe and respond as we do because we know what to expect from them; we know what to do to get them to meet our needs. For this reason we seek interaction, intimacy, and friendship with those who believe and behave in ways that make sense to us, and with whom we know what to do to get our needs met. Since our beliefs and behaviors were shaped by the world we grew up in, and we establish relationships with people we understand, we have a strong tendency to recreate that world as an adult, maintaining the culture, position, and parenting styles we are familiar with. This is the world that makes sense to us at the deepest levels, and at those levels we accept it as the real world and we are deeply affected by its values, beliefs, and practices. Others who are not from the small circle of our world can be relegated to the fringes of humanity; they can become "them" while we are "us."

Adjustment

We spend a great deal of time and effort establishing a life made up of the people, job, house, and community that meet our needs. Once these are in place and we are confident in our ability to get our needs met, our world is functional and we are secure. And then something changes. Death, divorce, disability, lay-off, promotion, geographic/cultural relocation, and any number of other things can remove elements from the world that people depend on to meet their needs. These unmet needs generate feelings that may not have been experienced for a long time, and the circumstances surrounding the change can produce an array of negative feelings, including insecurity, stress, anxiety, or grief. In order to remain functional the person is required to adjust, to begin again and put all of the pieces back into place and construct a new world that again meets his or her needs. No one escapes having to adjust to changes in life and the faster life changes the more we must adjust. But behavior is locked into physical structures in the brain so there is a limit to how fast we can change, and the world around us is changing faster all the time. Cultural diversity, economic necessity, technology, scientific and medical innovation, government policy, war, genocide, migration—all represent areas of rapid change whose impact often leaves many struggling to cope in a world they do not understand. The older we get the more difficult adjustment becomes, and if we are unable to accomplish it we may spend the remainder of our lives alienated in loneliness, bitterness, intolerance, despair, or even in chronic grief. One of the major challenges of providing health care services to patients and family members is their active struggle to adjust to issues caused by the loss of health, physical ability, body image, employment, or the partial or complete loss of a loved one. This struggle to adjust can result in sorrow, resentment, anger, even rage—which is at times misdirected at health care practitioners.

DYSFUNCTION

Beliefs and behaviors that succeed in getting needs reasonably well met are **functional** beliefs. The development of these is a long, complex process that locks the beliefs into a physical brain structure that resists change, thus limiting the speed of adjustment. Remaining functional in today's ever-changing world requires a rate of adjustment that stretches the limits of human adaptability. This may turn out to be the major social issue of our time, and health care practitioners must be aware of its impact in their own lives and in the lives of their clients. Beliefs and behaviors that do not succeed in getting needs reasonably well met are **dysfunctional** beliefs. These may be the result of growing up under the influence of a negative parenting style, or of the inability or refusal to make the adjustments necessary to maintain effective functioning. As dysfunction grows, needs are more and more unfulfilled. As those needs continue to be unfulfilled they grow increasingly stronger until they create powerful feelings that can in themselves increase dysfunction. Not feeling safe and secure can drive feelings of mistrust, insecurity, and suspicion; not being loved can fuel desperation, doubt, and despair; lack of acceptance can result in loneliness and resentment; and lack of respect can lead to feelings of inferiority. We process these feelings with self-talk that flows from our beliefs, and if our beliefs are dysfunctional the behaviors that result will be dysfunctional and our needs will continue to be unmet. One of the major challenges of development is in taking the simple beliefs we arrive at adulthood with and changing them into more mature beliefs as we experience more and more of the changes and ambiguities of life. In order to do this we must accept our feelings and take responsibility for our emotions and actions, and the key to all of this lies in what we believe.

Irrational Beliefs

Beliefs that do not allow us to get our needs met are dysfunctional. That does not mean that the belief is inherently irrational. In a dysfunctional environment **rational** beliefs may in fact be dysfunctional. To be abnormal in an abnormal situation is normal. For a child no belief is irrational. Children simply learn what they need to survive in the world they are born into. The problem develops when they leave that small world and enter the larger world of adulthood. Beliefs and behaviors that were necessary in the small world of their childhood may set them up for dysfunction in the larger adult world. There is an almost unlimited supply of **irrational** beliefs; some of the more common are:

"I should always keep complete control over myself and others."
Everyone struggles and no one has the ability to completely control themselves, nor the ability or right to control others.

"I should never feel inadequate, vulnerable, or sad."
You cannot remain human and escape human frailty or emotions. Everyone feels bad sometimes.

"Things are either right or wrong, good or bad, there is nothing in between."
To merely observe that nearly everything is some shade of gray would be to miss the point. Right and wrong are judgments that we have little right to make. While we must have a set of values to guide our behavior, we find it all too easy to condemn others who don't live up to our ideas of what should be. There is nothing more harmful than condemnation, and it usually makes a much stronger statement about the one doing the condemning than it does about the one being condemned.

"Life should be easy, what I want should be given to me."
Life does not follow our ideas of what "should" be. It is not easy and never comes with a guarantee. No one, including you, is so special as to deserve everything they want, or so smart that they always know what is best for them.

"I should always feel good, I should be happy, confident, and in control."
No one is always happy or confident or in control. We are all just human and as such are vulnerable and conflicted.

"People who love each other should never fight."
Caring about people gives them a great deal of power over you and your emotions. If you don't care enough about someone for them to have the power to make you angry, they most likely don't have the power to make you happy. People who care about each other almost always go through a very emotional learning and adjusting period before they establish the ground rules and understandings that enable them to live in relative harmony. It's like two rivers meeting to churn and boil before becoming an even more powerful one.

"I cannot be alone; if I am alone, I feel empty and miserable."
Learning to be alone is invaluable. We all extend ourselves outward, reaching to and for others, but we must have a center to reach out from. Creating a stable center—knowing who you are, learning to stand on your own, being OK alone—is a necessary foundation for relationships with others. Without that foundation we can become weak and dependent and too easily end up playing roles that trap us and isolate us from our own identities. The idea that we will be miserable if we are alone causes us to impose that belief on ourselves rather than taking the opportunity to enjoy and learn from the solitude.

"Others should be the way I think they should be."
A tremendous number of factors combine over the years of a lifetime and the centuries of a culture to create the person in front of you. It is arrogant to insist that they measure up to some arbitrary standard that you create.

"I should never fail or make a mistake."
We are human. Humans are imperfect. Everyone fails, everyone makes mistakes. These are opportunities for growth. The main damage comes usually not from the mistake, but from self-condemnation and defeat. It does no good to kick yourself. The only productive response when you find yourself on the ground is to

think about how you got there and how not to make the same mistake again. Then get back on your feet and start over. Those who are ultimately successful are not the ones who are too strong to fall, rather they are the ones who simply refuse to quit and will always get up one more time than they fall down. As Muhammad Ali once said "Inside of a ring or out, ain't nothing wrong with going down. It's staying down that's wrong."

"No one will like me or love me if they find out I'm weak or imperfect."

People may respect or even be in awe of strength and perfection, but friendship and love are given to those they can identify with, who seem most like themselves. We find a definite pleasure in discovering that some "great" person has weaknesses or flaws just like us. Try to be a good person, not a perfect person. You don't have to be better than others in order to be as good as them. Who you are is the only person you can be, and if you allow it to be it is a wonderful thing, far better than anyone you could pretend to be.

"My worth as a person depends on what I accomplish or on how I look."

In our culture accomplishments and looks are valuable things, but if you're not enough without them, you'll never be enough with them. We confuse value and worth. A baby has no practical value, it cannot produce anything or help anyone, yet it has unlimited worth. We don't outgrow that worth and it cannot be measured, and certainly not contained by such surface things as accomplishments or looks. Such things are only ways in which we establish status, a very primitive drive. Accomplishments and beauty are shallow and those who rely on them for their self-worth are forever doomed to live on the surface, barely aware of their own existence. The qualities and abilities that make us truly human are much deeper and more complex.

"I must have approval from everyone."

No one can please everyone. No matter what you believe, there will always be those who disagree, and those who strongly disagree. No matter what you do, some will be displeased. Trying to please everyone usually ends up pleasing no one, least of all your self. You can give and give right up to the limit of your resources and ability, and when you reach that limit there will always be those who condemn you for what you cannot do rather than praise you for what you have done. Other people are usually much more content if you establish limits and hold to them. Then they know what to expect from you, and in time come to accept what you have to give rather than to continually push to get more.

"If something goes wrong, it proves to everyone that I am worthless."

Doubt, guilt, and inferiority create a deep sense of worthlessness, and to someone who feels worthless there is little more frightening than the prospect of a failure that will display their inferiority to the world. When something goes wrong it is necessary for them to hide it, deny it, blame it on someone else—anything to keep from being convicted by it. It is almost pointless to say to that person that everyone makes mistakes, everyone fails sometime, and that the only sensible thing to do is accept it and try to figure out how it went wrong and where to go from here.

"People who do bad things are bad people and they should be blamed and punished."

People do bad things, sometimes by mistake, sometimes out of weakness, sometimes out of malevolence. Most have an inner voice that pushes them to do the right and avoid the wrong, and doing bad things does not make them bad people. While we do have to protect ourselves from the small group who seem to lack that voice, we cannot simply throw away everyone who makes a mistake. It is from our mistakes that we learn, and people do have a right to be wrong. We are in danger of becoming a society of "I should never fail or make a mistake."

"Being happy depends on the things a person gets or how important they are."

Happiness comes from the quality of personal relationships. Possessions and importance are issues of status on the primitive reptilian level and cannot satisfy our emotional needs for love, acceptance, or esteem, or free us to be ourselves. Only our relationships with other people can satisfy those needs and bring us any lasting happiness or satisfaction.

Defense Mechanisms

In the larger world, irrational beliefs such as those described above produce dysfunctional behavior that cannot meet our needs. As these unmet needs grow stronger the beliefs that do not meet them are under constant pressure. If the beliefs are to be kept unchanged they must be defended by creating mechanisms to keep them in place. These defense mechanisms block adjustment, because with them we can believe and do whatever we want without being responsible for it. If I am not responsible for it I can not change it. As we move through our day, self-talk continually emerges from our appraisal of each situation. That **appraisal** is powered by our beliefs, and it is the way we process our feelings and transform them into specific emotions designed to power the actions we have determined are most likely to get our needs met. These actions either influence others to meet our needs or they do not. If our actions too frequently fail at the job they were designed for, getting our needs met, the needs grow and fuel the production of neurotransmitters that create powerful feelings driving us to continue trying to meet the needs. But our behaviors can be locked into dysfunctional repetitive patterns by irrational beliefs. This presents our belief system with a new issue to ponder. Why can I not get my needs met? There are two basic responses to that question: taking personal responsibility, which leads to adjustment; and not taking personal responsibility, which leaves you with the problem of explaining why you cannot get your needs met. The effort to avoid this and the explanations that are manufactured are called defense mechanisms. **Defense mechanisms** function to insulate us from our feelings or from the responsibility for our feelings; they block our actions or shield us from the responsibility for our actions; and they are incorporated into our belief systems, where they shape our perceptions and alter our reality to fit into our picture of it. Some of the more common defense mechanisms are

Repression: Burying the memory of emotional or physical trauma in the unconscious. If the conscious mind doesn't know that it ever happened it doesn't have to find a way to cope with it. This can happen at any age, but is most necessary for children, who have not yet developed the mental abilities they need to understand and cope. The downside of repression is that by not coping with trauma the buried feelings remain alive and unchanged, and can emerge unbidden from the unconscious mind to drive bewildering and self-defeating behaviors.

Denial of reality: Protecting yourself from the consequences of an unpleasant reality by acting as if it were not real. The young mother who clearly understands the harsh realities of being a single mother on her own may choose not to believe her daughter's report of sexual abuse by her new step-father.

Fantasy: Building "air castles." Compensating for feelings of inadequacy or inferiority by investing emotion in imaginary abilities, achievements, or plans, but never working to make any of those a reality.

Reaction formation: Convincing yourself and others that you don't feel and want the things you do, and keeping yourself from acting on your feelings, by building an exaggerated identity around opposing values and condemning others who act like you want to.

Projection: Blaming others for your feelings or actions, or assuming that someone else is guilty because you would do or would like to do what you think they did.

Displacement: Taking out your feelings, usually anger, on someone who isn't as dangerous as the person who got you mad.

Emotional insulation: Giving up and not trying to get your needs met, becoming numb, or adopting a "who cares? It (he/she) wasn't worth the effort anyway" attitude to keep from getting hurt or disappointed.

Intellectualization: Coming up with strong, logical, self-convincing reasons to explain why things are the way they are in order to keep from being hurt by them. "All men are pigs, so of course every man I pick is one."

Rationalization: Attempting to prove logically that negative behavior is rational and justifiable and thus worthy of self- and social approval, for example, "They had it coming."

Regression: Retreating backward down the emotional maturity ladder to use less mature feelings and actions, developed at an earlier age, when you don't know what to do.

Identification: Making up for your own feelings of inferiority or inadequacy and feeling better about yourself by connecting yourself to someone or something that you or others admire, and taking your self-worth and identity from that person or organization.

Compensation: Making up for weaknesses in one area by becoming very strong in another way. Or making up for unmet needs by taking too much of things that you can get, such as overeating when you're lonely.

Acting out: Reducing the pressure caused by forbidden or dangerous feelings by allowing them to flow directly into actions; "I did not plan it, it just happened."

Undoing: Doing something good to make up for having done something bad, usually after having acted out. But flowers and promises and good behavior last only so long, and there are only so many times you can put your world back together again. After a while, others grow tired of your excuses and don't believe your promises any more than you do.

Everyone, or at the very least almost everyone, has used defense mechanisms at some point in their life. Beliefs, emotions, and actions are programmed into the physical structure of the brain and there is an investment of years of experience and growth into that structure. We will always use the existing structure first, and only grow or program a new one if it consistently fails to meet our needs. Defense mechanisms allow us to bend the world to fit into our structures, so that we do not have to change. But they do not get our needs met, and as those needs grow we must commit more and more energy into maintaining our defenses. This takes us further and further into isolation, self-absorption, and despair. In order to avoid that situation we must take responsibility for ourselves, drop our defenses, and put in the hard work it takes to adjust.

ADJUSTING

We arrive at adulthood with the beliefs, emotions, and actions that we learned in the world of our childhood. But the world we grew up in is seldom the one we are required to make our way in as adults, and we can find ourselves drifting with no sense of how to construct a fulfilling life, one that meets our needs. Or we find a compass and work our way to a fulfilling life, and then change, that constant reality of the modern world, thrusts us into someplace or with someone new, and once more we have to adjust. Maintaining a fulfilling life requires continual **adjustment**.

Self-Talk

If our beliefs are rational they will result in productive self-talk, and in time we will make any adjustments necessary; but if our beliefs are irrational they will result in unproductive self-talk that reflects the defense mechanisms blocking us from adjusting. In the end, the greatest asset or liability we have is what we believe, and the key to understanding what we believe is in listening to what we are saying to ourselves—our self-talk. Our willingness to say negative things to ourselves about ourselves is one of the most damaging things we can do. Changing negative self-statements to positive ones is an important step toward adjustment. Listen to yourself for statements that reflect negative beliefs and change them to statements that reflect positive ones. There are typical kinds of self-talk at each need or moral level. Some examples are:

Physical/power
- *Negative self-talk*: I am worthless. I am not lovable, important, or powerful. It isn't possible or it isn't safe to get close to others, trust them, or to ask for help. I do not deserve to be helped. What I do does not count if I have to ask for help; I will die or survive alone.
- *Positive self-talk*: I am worthy. I am loved and I belong here and deserve care. It is OK to ask for what I need. I can trust and rely on others. I am not alone.

Safety and security/deals
- *Negative self-talk*: I am not powerful. I deserve to die or I will live in spite of them. It is all my fault or it is all their fault. I'll be good or I'll be bad. Big people get to hurt little people. I will never hurt other people or I will always hurt other people. I will not feel or I will feel intensely. I am alone.
- *Positive self-talk*: It is OK to be me. I am a good person. I learn from my mistakes and continually grow more competent and capable.

Love/good boy
- *Negative self-talk*: I am not lovable and I do not deserve attention. I hate myself and I will humiliate myself and show everyone that I am no good. If others like me there is something wrong with them. I must be perfect. I must be better than others to be as good as them.
- *Positive self-talk*: I am lovable, capable, and I can be powerful. I can know what I need and it is OK to ask for what I need. I continually grow more responsible and competent.

Belonging/rules
- *Negative self-talk*: If other people know me they will not like me. I reject myself. I do not know who I am or what is right. I must please other people; I must be what they say I should be. I am what I do. Powerful people get what they want. I cannot question authority. Love and friendship obligate me and are too costly. I keep my distance emotionally. I do not trust others; I will run away and blame them.
- *Positive self-talk*: I can be both separate and connected, deciding when to be dependent or independent. I know who I am. I accept myself. If other people know me, they will like me.

Esteem/social contracts
- *Negative self-talk*: I am not worthy of respect, I do not respect myself. Other people are right not to listen to me. I have nothing of value to say.
- *Positive self-talk*: I am worthy of respect, I respect myself. It is OK to ask why or to question authority. People will listen to me.

Self actualization/individual conscience There is little or no negative self-talk at this level.
- *Positive self-talk*: We are all in this together. We all struggle with life and generally do the best we can. People have a right to make mistakes. People are what really matters. I have a responsibility to my fellow humans and to life. Life is good.

Since beliefs and behaviors are locked into physical brain structure it is always far easier initially to use them even if they do not fit the reality our new world and to blame our new world for not meeting our needs. Adjustment is blocked by irrational beliefs, which result in negative self-talk that powers defense mechanisms. To move beyond this impasse it does no good to try to resolve problems externally. The problems after all were caused by our own beliefs, self-talk, and defenses and these are all we have to try to solve them with. It is much more productive to work on solutions to negative self-talk and beliefs. These solutions require change, becoming something you are not, yet.

Change

Change requires growth, new connections in the brain creating new abilities. In childhood this kind of growth is stimulated by interactions with the environment for which the child has no responsibility. Who we are when we enter the adult world is not our fault, but as adults we must become responsible for directing our own growth. Who I will be tomorrow is my responsibility. But how do I guide myself to become something I am not? How can I conceive of something that is not? The answer is in the abstract abilities of the neocortex of the brain. By the time we are adults the neocortex is well enough developed to conceive of what should be and to push us to become that. Imagination is the path to the future. But the imaginings must be grounded in knowledge; they must be realistic. Read all you can until you come to understand as well as possible what it is you want to become. Identify the irrational beliefs, negative self-talk, and defense mechanisms you are using and stop using them. At first this may mean simply stopping in the middle of saying something negative to yourself or in the middle of saying or doing something directed at someone else, but eventually you will be able to substitute the negative self-talk with the positive self-talk and actions that you want to be able to do. Watch other people who seem to be capable of doing what you desire. Then imagine yourself in specific situations responding as you would like to be able to respond. Build the image until it becomes a world in your mind and you feel it to be true. The better you can see it and feel it, the easier it will be to become it. Now go out and try to do it. And do not be discouraged when you cannot. Seeing something in your imagination is one thing, doing it is something else. There are very real physical structures in your brain locking you into your old responses. If you are working to challenge irrational beliefs, overcome defense mechanisms, and change your life, *do not give up. Do not give up. Do not give up. Do not give up. Do not give up. Do not give up. Please. Do Not Give Up.* The more you imagine and the more you try the faster your brain figures out what it is you are trying to do and what connections are necessary to make it work. This is a complex process and you should expect it to take several months at least. Those who are ultimately successful are not the smartest, strongest, or the fastest; they are just stubborn enough to keep trying. No matter if others are tired of your ups and downs, no matter if you are tired of your ups and downs, just keep getting up every time you fall and keep putting one foot in front of the other. Watch others who can do it, imagine yourself doing it, keep trying to do it. One day you will be surprised to discover that you are doing it without having to try. New connections will have grown, creating new abilities. The longer you continue to use the new connections the more efficient and effective they will become, until those around you accept this new you, and until, finally, you do too.

Stress

But always remember, stress drives you backward. Growing and using new pathways and new connections does not automatically disconnect the old ones. If they are unused for long enough the old connections may deteriorate and break down, but they are well established and the process can take years, perhaps decades. In the meantime you must always be aware that they still exist, and that they will still work. Stress can drive you back to those earlier patterns, even after years of living a new life. **Stress** is caused by changes that require more effort. Marriage, conflict, money problems, divorce, having children, being promoted, changing jobs or adding more responsibilities to your existing job, relocation, accidents, illness, disability, death—any of these can cause stress, and we need to understand how we respond to it. There are four stages in **stress reaction**: alarm and mobilization, resistance, decompensation, and disintegration.

The Stress Reaction

Stage 1: Alarm and Mobilization. People respond to a stressor by focusing their attention on it, gathering their resources, and working harder. In this stage people often are extremely productive, they push themselves and may be able to withstand or accomplish far more than they would have believed possible. But this cannot last forever.

Stage 2: Resistance. If the stress is short-lived people quickly return to normal. But if the stress continues for too long they begin to get tired and have to find a way to live with the stress and make the extra effort that it takes to just keep going. Their strength and attention is focused on what they have to do to and they have little left for anyone around them. In this stage people regress to earlier, less mature coping strategies and become so preoccupied with the effort to keep things together that they have little emotional strength left for anyone around them and may become impatient, intolerant, and selfish.

Stage 3: Decompensation. If the stress continues, people become exhausted and cannot keep going. This is a time of physical, emotional, or mental collapse and any semblance of normal functioning is impossible. This is a time to stop trying, get away from the stress, and rest.

Stage 4: Disintegration. If it isn't possible to get away from or resolve the stress, people will completely break down, physically, mentally, or emotionally. It may not be possible to return to normal once disintegration has happened; death is common.

From the resistance stage onward, people are pushed back to earlier coping strategies. If these were dysfunctional, they can become a stranger to those around them. "I do not even know who you are any more" is an enormous red flag. Within a few days to weeks a person can tear apart a world that has taken them years to build.

A relationship may be strong enough to withstand one or more of these episodes, but there are only so many times that a world can be rebuilt before it falls apart forever. If you have overcome dysfunction in your life by putting in the time and effort to build new, more productive pathways you must always be aware that stress can drive you backward and take your world away. When under significant stress it is of the utmost importance that you just do not act. You cannot resolve conflicts, discipline your child, or make important decisions. In this condition the last thing you may want to do is stop and walk away, but anything you do will most likely only make things worse. There will be another day, and you can address issues on that day without the risk of hurting those you love most in the world.

SUMMARY

Personality traits, beliefs, emotions, and actions are all developed to make it possible for us to meet our needs in the world in which they develop. We spend a great deal of time and effort building a life that reflects the world of our childhood and in which we understand how to meet our needs, but we can never be in complete control of the world we create. People treat us in ways and we act in ways and discover things that challenge our self- and world concepts. We must make continual minor adjustments to keep a clear perspective on who we are so that we can know what to do. Dreams may be instrumental in making these adjustments. But minor adjustments are not always enough. Major changes can take place. Migration places the person in a completely different world that quite often makes no sense to them. Death, incapacitation, divorce, job loss, and innumerable other things can completely remove elements from a person's world that he or she depended on to meet their needs. When these things happen, people must adjust in a major way to rebuild a functional world and to find a way to get their needs met.

Dysfunction can grow at many points. If people are not able to establish an adult world that meets their needs, if they cannot make the continuous minor adjustments to keep a functional world balanced, or make the major adjustments necessary to re-build a shattered world, their needs will not be met. Unmet needs grow more and more powerful and produce demanding feelings. The belief system is the pivotal element in turning these feelings into either productive, need-meeting behaviors or into unproductive behaviors that cannot meet needs. Rational beliefs can be identified by positive self-talk and they produce productive behaviors. Irrational beliefs can be identified by negative self-talk and they produce unproductive behavior. Changing unproductive behavior to productive behavior and achieving adjustment can be accomplished by identifying and challenging irrational beliefs and changing negative self-talk to positive. This will create the ability to stop using the unproductive behavior. The next step is to find out what productive behavior looks like, imagine doing it, and then try to do it. Do not expect to be good at it at first, but practice makes perfect, and the more you try the faster the brain connections will grow until new abilities are created that can turn a dysfunctional world functional.

Be aware of stress. Stress drives a person backward to less mature patterns of beliefs, emotions, and actions and can drive a functional world back into dysfunction. Under significant stress do not attempt to make major decisions, resolve conflicts, or discipline children. Walk away and resist the temptation to destroy the new world you have built. You can deal with the issues when you are once again more the person you want to be and less the person you used to be.

APPLICATION SKILL

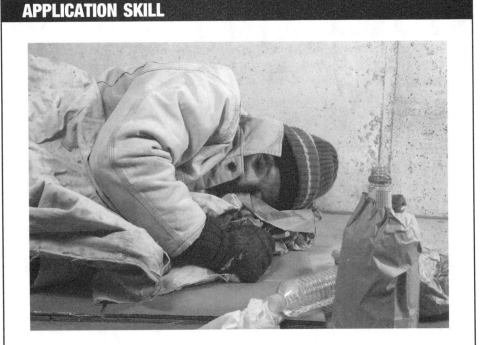

Ask

You have really looked at the person in front of you. You have allowed yourself to feel your response to them but have not judged them. You have listened attentively. Now it is time to ask for the information and understanding that you need.

A 40-year-old, drug-addicted resident of the streets is admitted to your hospital with an abscess on his thigh at an injection site. A surgeon performs an incision and drainage and places him on IV antibiotics for 14 days to clear the infection. As the patient withdraws from the drugs he becomes increasingly agitated, angry, rude, and demanding of the staff. On his third day he leaves the hospital, against medical advice (AMA). Nearly two weeks later he returns to the hospital, his thigh significantly worse. The surgeon again performs an incision and drainage and places him on two weeks of IV antibiotics. He again leaves

APPLICATION SKILL (continued)

against medical advice after only a few days. On his third admission the infection is severe, possibly into the thigh bone itself. A third incision and drainage is performed and he is again placed on a two-week regimen of IV antibiotics. If he leaves again the overwhelming likelihood is that when he returns his leg will have to be amputated at the hip. The pattern begins to be repeated and he becomes increasingly agitated, angry, and rude with the staff as he withdraws from the drugs. It is obvious that he is close to leaving again against medical advice before the infection is cleared. What do you do?

Most people have comfort zones and do not often or easily move beyond their boundaries. Health care professionals cannot afford to allow personal boundaries to limit their ability to provide effective health care; they must be able to do what is necessary. The drug-addicted resident of the streets in the above example is being driven by personal needs and fears. Accepting him as a person and listening openly without judgment creates the ability to ask direct questions about his addiction and the experience of withdrawal, and it creates the opportunity for him to listen to an explanation of the consequences of his choices. Do not hesitate, simply ask and try to understand. Understanding opens the possibility of empathy, of being able to consider what you would feel in his place. Empathy motivates the effort to explore every possibility, inside and outside of the box, in the effort to find a solution.

CONCEPT REVIEW

1. **Functional** behaviors influence others in our environment to respond in such a way as to meet our needs. **Dysfunctional** behaviors produce a response in others that does not meet our needs.

2. Separations between people begin with differences in genetic predispositions but are magnified by the beliefs and behaviors taught by parents, position, and culture.

3. Safety and security come from knowing what to do. If I have no doubt about my ability to meet my physical needs, stay safe and secure, give and receive love, be accepted, and respected I am secure and comfortable in my surroundings. For this reason I have a strong tendency to recreate the world of my childhood as an adult, maintaining the culture, position, and parenting styles I am familiar with and seeking interaction, intimacy, and friendship with those who believe and behave in ways that make sense to me.

4. Others who are not from my world can be relegated to the fringes of humanity; they can become "them" while we are "us." The word that describes this is **ethnocentrism**, the belief that your culture's values, beliefs, and practices are right, which makes others who do not share those values, beliefs, and practices wrong.

5. Any number of other things can remove elements from the world that a person depends on to meet their needs. In order to remain functional the person is required to **adjust**; to put the pieces back into place and construct a new world that again meets their needs.

6. **Rational** beliefs are functional, as they lead to positive self-talk that promotes adjustment. **Irrational** beliefs are dysfunctional, as they lead to negative self-talk that promotes defense mechanisms which block adjustment.

7. **Dysfunctional** behaviors that do not meet our needs can be locked into repetitive patterns by irrational beliefs, and the belief system is brought into question by the individual who has to deal with the question: "Why can I not get my needs met?" Efforts to avoid this question or explanations manufactured to evade personal responsibility for it are called defense mechanisms.

8. Self-talk continually emerges from our appraisal of each situation as we move through our day. That **appraisal** is powered by our beliefs, and it is the way we processes our feelings and transform them into specific emotions designed to power the actions we have determined most likely to get our needs met. The part of this process we can become immediately aware of is our self-talk which is an open window into our beliefs.

9. Becoming aware of negative self-talk, irrational beliefs, and defense mechanisms enables a person to identify when they are using them and choose not to.

10. Becoming aware of positive self-talk and rational beliefs allows a person to practice using them in their imagination and to identify and try to perform behaviors based on them.

11. The more you imagine and the more you try the faster your brain figures out what you are trying to do and what connections are necessary to make it work. One day you will be surprised to discover that you are doing it without having to try. New connections will have grown, creating new abilities. The longer you continue to use the new connections the more efficient and effective they will become.

12. If you have overcome dysfunction in your life by putting in the time and effort to build new, more productive pathways you must always be aware that stress can drive you back to using the old, dysfunctional ones. When under significant stress it is of the utmost importance that you just do not act. You cannot resolve conflicts, discipline your child, or make important decisions. In this condition the last thing you may want to do is stop and walk away, but anything you do will most likely only make things worse. There will be another day, and you can address issues on that day without the risk of hurting those you love.

REVIEW QUESTIONS

I.   Completion

Complete the following sentences.

1. New abilities created by new connections in the brain enable us to _____.

2. A belief that produces behaviors that systematically do not get needs met is a(n) _____ belief.

3. Self-talk flows from our beliefs and reflects our _____ of a situation.

4. The stage of the stress reaction in which a person's strength and attention is focused on what they have to do and during which they may become impatient, intolerant, and selfish is _____.

II.   Multiple Choice

Select the letter of the choice that best completes the statement.

5. A defense mechanism can allow us to avoid (choose all that apply)
   A. Change
   B. Responsibility
   C. Unacceptable behavior
   D. Unacceptable feelings

6. Safety and security come from
   A. Being protected by others
   B. Staying out of dangerous situations
   C. Knowing what to do
   D. Power

7. The goal of adjustment is
   A. Productivity
   B. To continue to get needs met
   C. To resolve problems
   D. To avoid stress

8. Behaviors that systematically fail to get needs met are
   A. Irrational
   B. Self-defeating
   C. Morally superior
   D. Dysfunctional

9. Once new brain connections are grown and unsuccessful behaviors are replaced with successful ones, the old connections in your brain
   A. Disconnect very quickly
   B. Are consistently disregarded in favor of the new connections
   C. Remain intact for years and can reassert themselves without warning, especially during stress
   D. Are no longer a factor in your life

III.   Matching

10. Match each term with its correct description.
    A. Repression
    B. Regression
    C. Denial of Reality
    D. Identification
    E. Fantasy
    F. Compensation
    G. Reaction Formation
    H. Acting out
    I. Projection
    J. Undoing
    K. Displacement
    L. Emotional Insulation
    M. Intellectualization
    N. Rationalization

_____ Attempting to prove to self and others that negative behavior is logical and justifiable and thus worthy of self- and social approval.

_____ Burying the memory of emotional or physical trauma in the unconscious.

_____ Protecting yourself from the consequences of unpleasant reality by acting as if it is not real.

_____ Convincing yourself and others that you don't feel and want the things you do, and keeping yourself from acting on your feelings, by building an exaggerated identity around opposing values and condemning others who act like you want to.

_____ Taking out your feelings, usually anger, on someone who isn't as dangerous as the person who made you mad.

_____ Compensating for feelings of inadequacy or inferiority by investing emotion in imaginary abilities, achievements, or plans, but never working to make any of those a reality.

_____ Giving up and not trying to get your needs met, becoming numb, or adopting a "who cares, it (he/she) wasn't worth the effort anyway" attitude to keep from getting hurt or disappointed.

_____ Making up for your own feelings of inferiority or inadequacy and feeling better about yourself by connecting yourself to someone or something that you or others admire and taking your self-worth and identity from that person or organization.

_____ Blaming others for your feelings or actions or assuming that someone else is guilty because you would do or would like to do what you think they did.

_____ Coming up with strong, logical, self-convincing reasons to explain why things are the way they are in order to keep from being hurt by them.

_____ Retreating backward down the emotional maturity ladder to use less mature feelings and actions, developed at an earlier age, when you don't know what to do.

_____ Doing something good to make up for having done something bad.

_____ Making up for weaknesses in one area by becoming very strong in another way. Or making up for unmet needs by taking too much of things that you can get, such as overeating when you're lonely.

_____ Reducing the pressure caused by forbidden or dangerous feelings by allowing them to flow directly into actions.

IV. Critical Thinking

11. Why is changing behavior a long and difficult process?

12. Why would someone living in the world today probably have to adjust more during their lifetime than someone living a few hundred years ago?

13. If beliefs are rooted in brain structure that is unconscious, how can we become aware of what we believe?

Section 2
The Provider

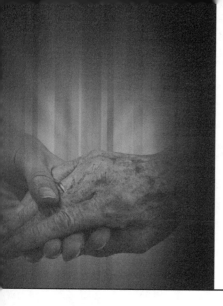

Chapter 5

Upon completion of this chapter you should be able to:

1. Define and contrast the characteristics of individualistic and collectivist cultures.
2. Define *ethnocentrism*.
3. Discuss the ethnocentric brain.
4. Define *territory*.
5. Define *status* and discuss its impact.
6. Define *ritual* and *aggression* as they apply to the defense of territory.
7. Discuss the causes and effects of "us" and "them."
8. Define *stigma*.
9. Define *bias*.
10. Define *stereotyping*.
11. Define *prejudice*.
12. Define *discrimination*.
13. List and discuss three types of stigma.
14. List and discuss nine types of bias.
15. List and discuss three types of discrimination.
16. Discuss the role of professional codes of ethics.
17. Define and discuss *professionalism*.
18. Discuss the role of education in reducing discrimination.
19. Discuss the role of employers in reducing discrimination.

KEY TERMS

individualistic culture	us	physical stigma
collectivistic culture	them	character stigma
multicultural	stigma	institutionalized
ethnocentrism	bias	discrimination
territory	stereotyping	personal discrimination
status	prejudice	internalized
ritual	discrimination	discrimination
aggression	tribal stigma	

Recognizing Your Own Beliefs

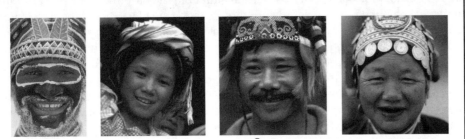
Accept

To accept another person is to receive them willingly, to respond favorably to them. To reject another person is to refuse to receive them willingly, to refuse to respond favorably to them. In the world around us there is a sea of difference. Age, lifestyle, race, nationality, language, culture, religion, status, appearance, values, ethics, ability, income, education, sexual orientation, interests, politics, and many, many other issues separate us. It is easy to care about, accept, and help those who are like us, whom we understand, especially when we see them as needing help through no fault of their own. But what of those whose personal or religious beliefs lead them to refuse the medical care we offer? What of those whose needs seem to us to be the product of their own choices? Do we find ourselves drawing away from a drug-addicted man with an infection at an injection site, a severely obese woman who compulsively eats sweets yet who has uncontrolled diabetes, a mentally ill person who seems to craftily plot ways to offend or manipulate us? What of the person who cries out for help and yet seems to thwart every effort we make to help them? What are the issues that we personally cannot understand? We all have limits to our ability to understand or accept. How do we move past those limitations and willingly receive those whom we cannot understand, and respond favorably to them?

INTRODUCTION

This chapter is about the biological basis of the drive to separate ourselves from and prejudge others, and the ways those appraisals shape our actions and can lead to discrimination, even if we are not consciously aware of it. It is also about how we can work to overcome our tendency toward bias in the delivery of health care.

Look for the physical structure of the brain responsible for creating and maintaining the natural processes that create patterns of stigma, bias, and stereotyping that in turn lead to prejudice and unjust discrimination. Look for the types of discrimination, and especially for how we can work to reduce bias and discrimination within the medical community and within ourselves.

After studying this chapter you should have a deeper appreciation for the power that bias exerts in the realm of human affairs and in your interactions with those to whom you have a health care responsibility. You should be aware of the dynamics of professionalism and the need to come to terms with your own limitations and your own beliefs.

FORMATION

The process of development is about learning how to meet our own needs. Since many of these needs are social needs, we must learn to interact with others in ways that motivate them to respond to us in ways that meet our needs. As adults we construct our world and fill it with others with whom we know what to do to elicit the required response. Others who are too different from us do not respond in the ways that we expect, so we gravitate toward those who are like us. That narrows our experiences, shapes our perceptions, and puts limits on our beliefs. Since our beliefs are responsible for our appraisals of each situation, they are the most powerful factor in perpetuating how we act toward others. In the small worlds of the past, where there was little change, childhood beliefs served people well; but in today's rapidly changing world we are constantly thrown into interactions with others who do not fit within the small world defined by our experiences and beliefs. If we are to respond appropriately to these others and avoid unfair discrimination, especially in the delivery of health care, we must become aware of the limitations of beliefs, both ours and theirs. We must look honestly at what we believe, why we believe it, and how that may be influencing the ways in which we deliver health care; until we become aware of these dynamics, we are ruled by them.

MULTICULTURALISM

Overpopulation, advances in international air travel, differences in economic opportunities, oppression, and war, among other things, have resulted in a rapid mix of cultures that can be radically different from each other.

At the far ends of this variation are individualistic and collectivist cultures. An **individualistic culture** values independence and personal responsibility. Individuals are given a great degree of autonomy and freedom but are seen as being responsible for meeting their own needs. There is little safety net with only very basic needs provided for should a person not be capable of providing for themselves. At the opposite end of the spectrum, a **collectivistic culture** values conformity to group values and rules, and there is considerable pressure on individuals to conform to shared beliefs and behaviors. There is a large safety net and a wide range of needs are provided for should a person not be capable of providing for themselves. Asian and socialist societies are generally collectivist, while western capitalistic societies are more individualistic.

Modern migration patterns move large numbers of individuals from collectivist to individualistic cultures, where they are often horrified at the chaos, crime, and social division that so often accompany increased individual freedom. Today's societies are a **multicultural** mix, with new arrivals every day. Each culture presents a unique environment with its own family structure, parenting beliefs, religion, value system, and many other elements. These variations result in very real differences in brain structure. Two adults raised in different families within one culture think and act differently; two adults raised in separate cultures can be so different as to make no sense to each other. Each is molded to a specific environment, accepting the beliefs and customs as right; and each relies on those beliefs and customs to guide them in situations that their parents could never have envisioned, living among others who think and behave in ways that can seem wrong. The word that describes this is **ethnocentrism**, the belief that your culture's values, beliefs, and practices are the right ones, which means that others who do not share those values, beliefs, and practices are wrong.

Because people within a particular group tend to share common values, habits, and customs, which they may not share with those from outside the group (Erlin, 1998), there is a strong tendency for ethnic groups to isolate themselves in pocket communities; or if the members of the group are spread throughout a new community, to interact primarily with each other. As most people do, they often feel more comfortable with those whom they perceive as similar to themselves, and favor members of their own group (Brewer, 1979). In our personal lives we are free to choose to remain isolated from those whose cultures we do not understand; but more and more, our professional lives make us responsible for their care. If we are to avoid responding to them in inappropriate ways and diminishing the quality of the care we provide, we must attempt to understand those from cultures different than our own, and we must recognize our own beliefs and take charge of our own behavior. The less we understand the feelings, responses, and behaviors of others, the more likely we are to interact inappropriately with them (Gardner, 1993).

THE ETHNOCENTRIC BRAIN

Ethnocentrism is nearly universal across every culture because, as with everything we feel, think, and do, it has a basis in the physical structure of the brain, and that structure is universal. The brain can be divided functionally into four layers: the brain stem, the reptilian complex, the limbic system, and the neocortex (Figure 1.9). The reptilian complex gets its name from the fact that it first appears in reptiles and is what separates them from fish, which have only a brain stem.

The point of developing a new layer of the brain is to gain more complex behaviors; the behaviors the reptile gained involved territory and status.

Amphibians and then reptiles evolved on strips of land adjacent to rivers. Such habitats provided only limited space and resources, and to successfully compete for these and survive required more complex behaviors. The reptilian layer of the brain developed as an adaptation to that pressure and made possible the behaviors involving territory and status.

Territory for a reptile or a human is that set of things they depend on to meet their needs. For a reptile that entails a physical area and everything in it. A good territory may include reliable sources of food, water, and shelter; places to hide; and safe ledges on which to lie in the sun. For a human, territory may include family, friends, home, job, career, achievements, and reputation. A good territory will fulfill needs that a poor territory will not. The reptile or person with the better territory has the higher **status** and is sought after and deferred to. Those with higher status are seen as more important and are given more rights and freedoms, including more right and freedom to mate and to live. A female reptile who will mate and lay eggs needs to lay them in the territory that will best ensure their survival. Reptile heaven—abundant food, water, and shelter—makes much better sense than barren rock and scrubby plants with little of any of those things. And reptile heaven will be the territory of the biggest, strongest, fastest, most aggressive reptile around, who is in a position to choose the most genetically sound (and therefore attractive) female. Biologically, this makes sense, since the biggest, strongest, fastest, most aggressive male genes are then given into the care of the most genetically sound female in order to produce offspring with the maximum chance for survival. With all that is at stake, territory is fiercely protected. A reptile whose territory is invaded is in danger of losing all that fulfills his needs and allows him to pass his genes on to future generations. The reptilian complex works the same in humans as it does in reptiles. Humans whose territory is invaded are also in danger of losing relationships, possessions, job, reputation, or other elements that they depend on to meet their needs. Just as reptiles do, people will instinctively defend their territory first with **ritual**—words, tone of voice, gestures, and body language—and if that fails, with

aggression—actions that negatively impact another's well-being. This behavior often operates in an unconscious manner, and people may not realize why they are responding as they do. People who strongly deny being prejudiced have been shown to discriminate against others (Bargh, 1994; Greenwald & Banaji, 1995). This discrimination is triggered when someone who is seen as not belonging comes into the neighborhood, engages with people, or competes for jobs. That person is invading a territory, and those who claim that territory as their own will defend it. Those we recognize as belonging in our territory are "**us**," and they are accepted and allowed. Those who do not belong in our territory are "**them**," and they are not accepted or allowed. A stranger invading our home, someone flirting with our spouse, a less-popular child sitting at our table, a foreigner competing for our job, an old car driving through a wealthy neighborhood—each is responded to as an invasion at a very primitive, reptilian level. Others who are not a part of our group and do not belong in our territory are not "us," they are "them." If this is true for those in our own culture who are not a part of our group, it is magnified for those who are not a part of our culture and whose beliefs and behaviors make no sense to us.

Status

While we respond most dramatically to those we identify as not belonging in our territory, the reptilian complex also directs our responses to those we identify as belonging in our territory but who have higher or lower status than we do. Higher status individuals have more power and are instinctively sought-after and deferred to by most, resisted by only a few. Most people instinctively grant them more rights and freedoms, and their lives are seen as more important. Leading politicians, movie stars, rock stars, some professional athletes, and supermodels are extreme examples, but the reptilian complex can also direct our approach to our supervisor and his or her approach to us. A supervisor-employee relationship in which both the supervisor and the employee accept the supervisor's right to act toward the employee in a harsh or demeaning manner that the supervisor would never accept from the employee is a primitive reptilian relationship. Power and control—being on top of things and capable of making things happen—raise a person's status. Lack of power and control—being in a dependent position—lowers a person's status. Anything that appreciably lowers a person's status will set us up to unconsciously react to that person in accordance with our perception of their status, not their needs. This is especially true if we perceive that they are to blame for their own situation. People are most willing to help others if they perceive that they are innocent victims with no control over their situation (Weiner, 1980). Substance abuse, obesity, HIV, mental illness, non-insulin-dependent diabetes, and chronic pain with no known cause, among others illnesses, are all situations in which the health care provider may blame the client for their own illness and, as a result, reduce the quality of care. As with other forms of discrimination, these processes function on an unconscious basis, and we are often unaware of our own motivations and behavior.

Stigma, Bias, and Discrimination

Anything that marks a person as being different in a way that makes them be perceived as lesser is a **stigma**. The difference may be that they are part of another group, or something that defines them as low in status within the group. Either way, the reptilian complex sets us up to respond to them according to their perceived status, rather than according to their needs, by creating a **bias**, a slant in how the person is perceived. Seeing a "black man" is different from seeing a man who is black, just as seeing a "gay man" is different from seeing a man who is gay. Seeing the person and then identifying traits enables us to respond to the person. However, seeing the traits first can trap us into responding to our *perception* of those traits without ever really seeing the person. **Stereotyping** is the belief that everyone who shares a specific trait has the same character. This leads to **prejudice**—prejudging the person based on the trait, which creates **discrimination**—a difference in how the person is treated. Discrimination in the delivery of health care is aggression; it is an action that negatively impacts the well-being of another.

Stigma based on a person's belonging to another group is called **tribal stigma**. There is a wide array of marks that can identify someone as belonging to a different group, including skin color, religion, language, and economic level.

Physical stigma and **character stigma** can lower a person's status within one's own group and are based on physical imperfection and character deficits.

Physical imperfections can include appearance, as well as disability and disease. Character deficits can include such things as dishonesty, disloyalty, and aggressiveness.

It is important to realize that stigmatizing people due to their possession of a specific trait has little to do with the person possessing the trait. The identification of the mark, the bias, and all that follows is the product of the belief system of the one who is doing the stigmatizing. Seeing a trait as undesirable most often has its foundation in beliefs created during childhood, and the feelings and thoughts those pathways and patterns of belief produce create the foundation for acting out those beliefs by disrespecting and discriminating against any person perceived to have the undesirable trait.

When biased beliefs are shared across a culture they can lead to **institutionalized discrimination**: reduced access to goods, services, and opportunities enforced openly by overt law or hidden in covert policy or practice. Institutionalized discrimination creates inequality in employment, education, and medical care. Biased individuals may practice **personal discrimination** when they deny another's access to goods, services, or opportunities. But perhaps the worst outcome of bias is **internalized discrimination**, in which a person raised as a victim of discrimination sees themselves as undeserving of the goods, services, or opportunities that others take for granted. In the end, internalized discrimination is possibly the most powerful of the forces that keep both overt and covert institutionalized discrimination in place.

There is an almost unlimited list of traits that different people are biased against. In the delivery of medical care some of the more common biases are

> *Socioeconomic* – based on the perception of the client's status in society
>
> *Age* – based on the age of the client
>
> *Substance abuse* – based on the addiction of the client to a drug or other substance
>
> *Ethnic* – based on the culture of the client
>
> *Racial* – based on the race of the client
>
> *Gender* – based on the sex of the client
>
> *HIV and AIDS* – based on the client's having the disease
>
> *Mental illness* – based on the mental impairment of the client
>
> *Obesity* – based on the weight of the client
>
> *Disability* – based on the disability of the client

What health care providers believe about the client is responsible for their appraisal of the client's situation and creates the emotion that motivates the way in which health care is delivered. If those beliefs include stigmatizing the client or blaming them for their own illness, a likely outcome is unfair discrimination in the delivery of health care, of which the health care provider may or may not be consciously aware.

In an effort to ensure that each client receives appropriate care, regardless of the perceptions or awareness of the provider, professional health care associations provide codes that present and interpret principles of professional ethics (Kasar & Clark, 2000). A health care practitioner who follows these principles can be assured of delivering adequate medical care. But deliberately following a set of rules in order to deliver adequate care is both superficial and artificial. It is a good safety net to use when we recognize that we are at risk of discriminating, but gaining knowledge and understanding is a better option. Knowledge and understanding can change the beliefs we use to appraise clients, and in so doing change the discriminating behavior itself. It is essential that health care providers recognize that biases exist in others and within themselves, attempt to understand differences, and eliminate their own biases (Erlin, 1998). To facilitate that development, health care education must balance traditional evidence-based knowledge with information that helps providers better understand themselves and their clients (Swick, 1998; Seroka, 1994). As important as initial education is, it is often not enough. Without ongoing attention and support, in time old patterns can reassert themselves. In order to keep the newly developed beliefs and appraisals functioning, providers need support and encouragement from the institutions that employ them, continuing educational programs and seminars, and ongoing opportunities to interact with clients and others who are different from them (Howell, Butler, Vincent, Watt-Watson, & Stearns, 2000). There is nothing more effective in reducing prejudice than coming to know some of "them" personally and finding out that they need and feel and want and love just like you. It is easy to be prejudiced at a distance. It is much harder when you have allowed yourself to know someone as a human being.

Professionalism

Stereotyping and prejudice can allow us to believe that we know someone and know what to expect from him or her without the bother of actually getting to know them. Even if you take the time and make the effort to get to know someone, it doesn't mean you are going to like them. But it is important to realize that just like stereotyping and prejudice, not liking someone is a personal judgment you have made based on your beliefs and a very small amount of information about that person. We are not infallible. We are only human and as such are all subject to the divisive mechanisms of the reptilian complex. Everyone is biased. Our brain is forever searching for patterns and for ways to organize and interpret information; it even makes animals and faces in the clouds. Just as we realize that the animal is not really in the cloud, we need to come to realize that the assessment we make of someone is not really that person. Professionalism is acting in the best interests of the client, with a commitment to deliver quality health care to all. That commitment is honored not in spite of the negative judgments we make of some clients, but because we do not make those judgments in the first place. The more we come to understand the workings of our own mind and come to grips with our own biases and limitations the easier it becomes to simply suspend judgment and provide quality health care.

SUMMARY

Beliefs are formed during our early development as we learn to meet our own needs. Unconsciously we accept these beliefs as reality and as adults work to construct a world made up of others who believe and act in ways that we understand. As effective as that might be in enabling us to get our needs met, it defines the small group of people whom we understand and interact with as "us" and all of the people outside of that group as "them." It also defines the relationships within the group in terms of how we interact with those having more and less status. All of this is locked into the nature and development of the brain. Ethnocentrism is an inherent characteristic of the primitive reptilian complex. This small, unconscious area of the brain provides powerful motivation to define our territory and our relative status within it and to defend that territory and position with both ritual and aggression (Sagan, 1977). That process leads to stigma, bias, stereotyping, prejudice, and unfair discrimination, which may become institutionalized in the law of the land and in the way generations of people are taught to think about others, and internalized in the way they learn to think about themselves. If we are to escape playing our part in this primitive legacy we must use the higher-level abilities of the neocortex to understand the process and to choose not to be controlled by it.

APPLICATION SKILL

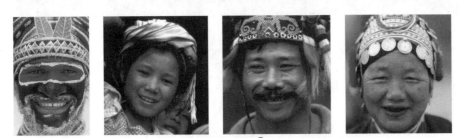

Photo from Plotnik. Introduction to Psychology (with Info TracA®)*, 7E. © 2005 Wadsworth, a part of Cengage Learning, Inc. Reproduced by permission.* www.cengage.com/permissions

Accept

We all have limits to our ability to understand or accept. How do we move past those limitations and willingly receive those whom we cannot understand, and respond favorably to them?

To accept another person is to receive them willingly, to respond favorably to them. To reject another person is to refuse to accept them, to refuse to receive them willingly or to respond favorably to them. Accept or reject; it is as simple as yes or no. Creation begins with yes. Stagnation begins with no. Are we trying to create, improve, or encourage something in them? Or are we trying to defend something in ourselves; in which case we will often discourage and destroy something in them. In the end we make a choice. That choice often has little to do with the other person standing before us; it is our choice made for our own reasons. Will we choose to defend us or to help them? One of the truly remarkable human ironies is that the more we choose ourselves, the less we become, and the more we choose others, the more we are. Accept the human being in front of you. You do not need to understand them. They are the product of their genetics and their world just as you are the product of yours. Relax and get on with doing the best you can to take care of what they need.

CONCEPT REVIEW

individualistic culture – Values independence and personal responsibility. Individuals are given a great degree of autonomy and freedom but are seen as being responsible for meeting their own needs. There is little safety net with only very basic needs provided for should a person not be capable of providing for themselves.

collectivist culture – Values conformity to group values and rules and there is considerable pressure on individuals to conform to shared beliefs and behaviors. There is a large safety net and a wide range of needs are provided for should a person not be capable of providing for themselves.

multiculturalism – Today's world is a multicultural mix with new arrivals every day bringing together people with widely different customs, values, and beliefs.

ethnocentrism – The belief that your culture's values, beliefs, and practices are the right ones, which makes others who do not share those values, beliefs, and practices wrong.

territory – The people, places, and things a person depends on to meet their needs; it may include family, friends, home, job, career, achievements, and reputation.

status – The person with the better territory, or more power within a mutual territory, has the higher status. They are afforded more rights and liberties and are sought after and deferred to.

ritual – Words, tone of voice, gestures, and body language instinctively used to defend territory or status against intrusion by someone who is seen as not belonging in the territory or deserving of the status.

aggression – Actions that negatively impact another's well-being used to defend territory.

us – Those we recognize as belonging in our territory and who are accepted and allowed.

them – Those we do not recognize as belonging in our territory and who are not accepted or allowed.

stigma – Anything that marks a person as being different in a way that makes them lesser.

bias – Perceiving a person as lesser, based on a stigma.

stereotyping – The belief that everyone who shares a specific stigma has the same character.

prejudice – Prejudging a person based on stereotyping. The assumption that a stigma tells you all you need to know in order to judge someone.

discrimination – A difference in how a person is treated based on a belief or prejudice rather than individual characteristics.

tribal stigma – A mark that identifies a person as belonging to another group. This may include things such as color, religion, language, accent, clothing, and economic level.

physical stigma – A physical imperfection that lowers a person's status within the group. This may include appearance as well as disability and disease.

character stigma – A perceived psychological or behavioral difference that lowers a person's status. Character stigmas may include such things as dishonesty, disloyalty, and aggressiveness.

institutionalized discrimination – When biased beliefs are shared across a culture and lead to a reduced access to goods, services, and opportunities and which is enforced openly by overt law or hidden in covert policy or practice.

personal discrimination – Personally denying another's access to goods, services, or opportunities based on bias.

internalized discrimination – The tendency of a person raised as a victim of discrimination to see themselves as undeserving of the same goods, services, or opportunities as others.

professionalism – Acting in the best interests of the client, with a commitment to deliver quality health care to all. That commitment is honored not in spite of the negative judgments we make of some clients, but because we do not make those judgments in the first place.

REVIEW QUESTIONS

I.   Completion

Complete the following sentences.

1. A deliberate act that harms someone else is _____.

2. Needs that are chronically unmet are _____.

3. The people, places, and things that we claim as our own and rely on to meet our needs are our _____.

4. A mark that identifies a person as belonging to a group seen as having lower status is a _____.

5. Treating people differently based on prejudice is _____.

II.   Multiple Choice

Select the letter of the choice that best completes the statement.

6. When facial expression, tone of voice, body language, and words are used to warn someone to leave our territory they are forms of
   A. Conflict
   B. Warning
   C. Aggression
   D. Ritual

7. Believing that your group has the right values, beliefs, and customs and that other groups do not is
   A. Discrimination
   B. Ethnocentrism
   C. Culture
   D. Bias

8. Power within a territory confers
   A. Responsibility
   B. Rights
   C. Status
   D. Freedom

9. Believing that everyone belonging to a group is alike is
   A. Stereotyping
   B. Prejudice
   C. Bias
   D. Realism

10. Laws of the past that allowed only white men to vote and own property are examples of
    A. Culture
    B. Institutionalized discrimination
    C. Internalized discrimination
    D. Bias

III.   Matching

Match each term with its correct description.

   A. Professionalism
   B. Prejudice
   C. Gender
   D. Tribal
   E. Physical

_____ Bias based on a person's belonging to another group.

_____ Bias based on disability.

_____ Working to provide quality health care to all.

_____ Bias based on the sex of the person.

IV.   Critical Thinking

11. How might you explain the tendency of black families to adopt light-skinned rather than dark-skinned black babies?

12. How does separating people into "us" and "them" affect the way we treat them?

13. Why does the medical profession need codes of ethics?

14. Why is simply trying to be professional not enough to eliminate our own biases and discrimination?

15. What is the role of the health care employer in eliminating bias and discrimination?

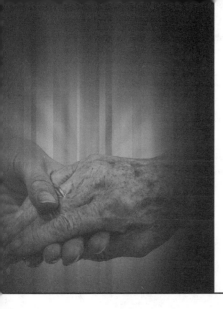

Chapter 6

Upon completion of this chapter you should be able to:

1. Define *social being*.
2. Define and discuss the nature of a social relationship.
3. Define and discuss the nature of a professional relationship.
4. Define *moral level* and discuss the impact on behavior.
5. Connect moral levels with levels of needs.
6. List and discuss six moral levels as they pertain to patient care.
7. Define *altruism*.
8. Define *skill*.
9. List and discuss 12 specific skills.

KEY TERMS

social beings	listen	empathy
professional relationship	ask	objectivity
moral levels	accept	behavioral modification
altruistic	encourage	stimulus
skills	assertiveness	behavior
look	anger management	response
wait	communication	

Being a Caregiver

APPLICATION SKILL

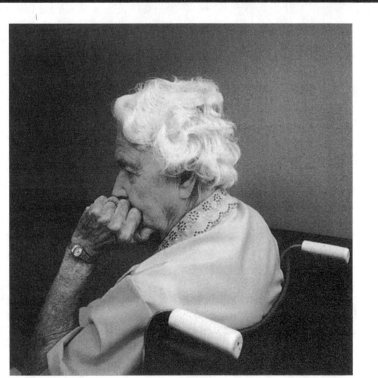

Encourage

You have really looked at the person in front of you. You have allowed yourself to feel your response without judging them. You have attentively listened and have asked for, and received, feedback. You have accepted them and are willing to work in their best interest, but they do not seem to have the will to try.

Scenario

The 78-year-old nursing home resident has the flu and she is giving up and dying. She has been a resident for just over a year and her family, who live a distance away, have stopped visiting on a regular basis. She is aware that she will never be able to live independently and she feels she's a burden. You are powerless to change the reality of her situation. How do you encourage her?

INTRODUCTION

This chapter is about providing care for others and offers explanations for the motivations behind at least some of this behavior. It also describes the balance that must be maintained in the give-and-take of need fulfillment in order for the caregiver to remain capable of delivering quality health care, and details several skill areas that can be developed to more effectively maintain this balance and fill the role of caregiver.

Look for the needs that drive individuals and the moral levels and limitations these needs motivate. Also look for the specific skills that can make you a better, more consistent caregiver.

After studying this section you should have some insight into the motivation to care for others, a clearer picture of how your personal life affects your professional life, and a better understanding of some specific skills that can help you cope with the stresses and demands of care-taking.

WHY DO WE CARE?

Humankind has a long history of caring for those in need. Early modern human and Neanderthal burials excavated from over 100,000 years ago reveal healed areas on bones that would have been devastating breaks and that would have required the care and support of others for the individual to have survived long enough to heal (Klein, 2003). What makes us willing to sacrifice our time, our resources, and sometimes even our lives for others?

A complete answer to that question certainly lies beyond the ability and scope of this book, but to attempt an answer let us expand the model of psychological functioning introduced in Chapter 2 (Figure 6.1).

Social Needs

We are **social beings**: many of our needs can only be met through relationships with others. The key to establishing and keeping productive relationships with others is that we must meet each other's needs. If our needs are not met well enough they will grow ever more powerful, making us more and more self-absorbed, and we will lose the ability to even see what someone else needs. This will render us unable to meet their needs and in time they will completely stop meeting ours. Meeting each other's needs is a give-and-take process. It is not necessary for all of our actions to meet the needs of another, nor for all of their actions to meet ours, but there must be a balance. The more one-sided the relationship becomes the more dysfunctional it is. How can we be safe if we can do nothing to prevent others from hurting us? How can

FIGURE 6.1

Expanded Model of Psychological Functioning.

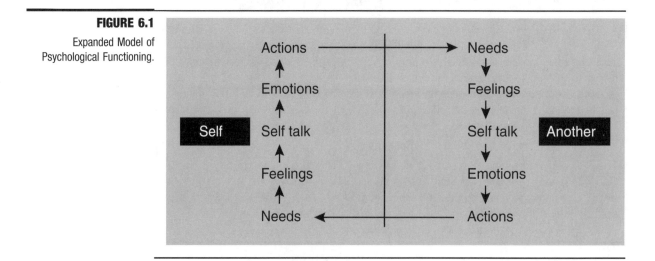

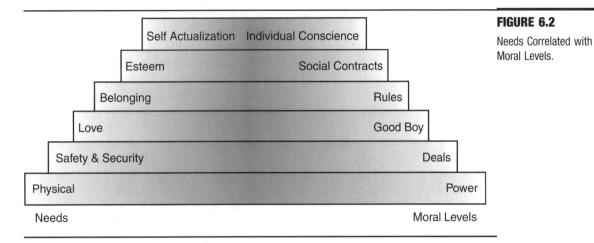

FIGURE 6.2

Needs Correlated with Moral Levels.

we be loved, accepted, or respected if others refuse to respond? In such relationships, the unmet needs grow and begin to drive increasing dissatisfaction and dysfunction.

So what makes a professional relationship possible? By definition, a **professional relationship** is one that exists to provide for the needs of the client, not the provider. Can one person, no matter what they are paid, consistently care for the needs of others while having their own needs go unmet? No, they cannot. As in any other unbalanced relationship, dissatisfaction and dysfunction will grow and it will reduce the quality of the care given. How can health care professionals consistently provide for the needs of others and meet their own needs in the process? First, you must ask what the provider needs. Maslow's hierarchy of needs (Figure 2.2) establishes multiple levels of needs that must be met in order. The lowest level need that is consistently unmet grows and motivates thoughts, emotions, and actions at that level. This motivation is the key to what Lawrence Kohlberg (1984) termed "moral levels." **Moral levels** are defined not by what we do, but by why we do it. As the lowest order need that is chronically unmet grows powerful it motivates behavior that can most often be defined and predicted by the morals at that level. As we saw in Chapter 2, each level of needs can be correlated with its own moral level (Figure 6.2).

Moral Motivation

The domination of physical needs motivates behavior at the power moral level. This level is completely self-serving; a person simply takes what they want, if they can. Compliance to rules is attained only by punishment and reward from those with more power. When functioning at this level a person is not motivated to care for another.

The domination of safety and security needs motivates behavior at the deals moral level. Deals are self-serving bargains that are made to get what a person wants, or to avoid what they do not want. When functioning at this level a person can be manipulative or coercive and is capable of being a "nice guy" in their manipulations, but is not capable of considering the needs of another before their own.

The domination of the need for love motivates behavior at the good boy/good girl moral level. When functioning at this level, a person is capable of great personal sacrifice if that sacrifice succeeds in getting appreciation and affection from others. If it does not, they can become bitter and vengeful. This produces an unpredictable and unstable level of care.

The domination of the need for belonging motivates behavior at the rules moral level. At this level a person is motivated by the rules operating in any given situation, which provide a pathway to acceptance and belonging. When functioning at this level a person is motivated by factors beyond the immediate interactions with a client. If the institution or peer group provides acceptance and appreciation, the provider is getting his or her needs met and can consistently deliver quality health care. If these reinforcements are not received the provider's needs are not met, and he or she can become increasingly alienated, thus decreasing the quality of care.

The domination of the need for esteem motivates behavior at the social contract moral level. Functioning at this level, providers are motivated by the needs of others and for the most good for the most people. They are not dependent on appreciation from clients, their peers, or the institution. If they perceive that they are doing what they should be doing and that they are helping others, this perception alone meets their need and they are able to consistently deliver quality health care.

For the few who develop to the level of self-actualization, needs are motivated by the principles of their individual conscience. These are principles such as fairness, equality, and justice. They have a deep empathy for people and love for mankind that are independent of the actions of others. They are capable of delivering unwavering quality health care, regardless of the situation.

It is vital to note that the providers' world is not limited to their professional relationships. If their needs are met well in their personal life they will be much more resilient to professional stresses. But if providers' needs are not met in their personal life, whether that is due to long-term realities, poor choices, or sudden changes, the longer this continues the more dependent the providers become on the nature of their professional relationships. Those include relationships with the institution they work for, their supervisor, peers, clients, and often their clients' families. If providers are not getting their needs met either in their personal or professional lives those needs will grow increasingly more powerful, centering them more and more on themselves, making it increasingly more difficult to see or feel what others need, and the delivery of health care will suffer.

Personality Traits of the Care Giver

The next issue that must be considered is the personality of the caregiver. As we saw in Chapter 2, individuals who score high on the personality trait of agreeableness are genuinely concerned for the welfare of others. These individuals are often **altruistic**, that is, willing to sacrifice their own needs for the good of another. A person who scores low on agreeableness is more concerned with his or her own needs and is generally unwilling to sacrifice them for the good of another. It makes intuitive sense that individuals who score high on the trait of agreeableness are more likely to seek a career of service to others and are more resilient in overcoming the stresses involved. But no one is an island, we are social beings. While our personality traits can make us more resilient, no one can continue to meet the needs of others if their own needs are chronically unmet. Ironically, a satisfying personal life is one of the most powerful resources for your professional life. The more whole we become as a person, the more we have to give to others.

SKILLS

As with any activity, providing care for others involves behaviors that must be learned. These activity related behaviors are **skills**. Each health care specialty has its own specific skill set, but there are also skill areas that are helpful in every specialty because they are helpful in dealing with people in general, and with the stresses involved in caregiving. Some of these skills have been mentioned in the application section of each chapter. The following is a somewhat deeper look.

Skill 1: Look

To **look** at another person is our primary method of gathering information about them. Human DNA provides a plan for the construction of an extensive information-processing apparatus in the brain that almost instantly interprets a wealth of information about another person. Facial expression and coloration, body position and posture, arm position, eye contact and content, clothing—not just what is worn but how it is worn—grooming, and much more. Every piece is fit into every other piece until they merge in us as an intuitive feeling that tells us how and sometimes whether to approach a person. To gather and reason through all of that information could take hours or days, but it is all available in the time it takes to walk across a room. Do not glance at a patient, look at them. See them. Many specialties in health care teach specific observational skills, but Mother Nature has endowed us with an innate ability that can provide a foundation stone for every other skill we may possess. All we have to do to access that ability is to look.

Skill 2: Wait

The unconscious mind is aware of its limitations. It is always looking to the conscious mind for direction. That is the reason that changing from negative self-talk to positive self-talk produces more positive emotions. As stated in Chapter 2, our beliefs shape our appraisal of a situation and that appraisal emerges as self-talk. We must not allow our beliefs to produce self-talk that results in unprofessional, biased behavior. We must **wait** and delay our reaction long enough to allow ourselves to act productively. By shaping what we say to ourselves in the all-important first moments of an interaction, we can avoid hasty appraisals and take the time we need to understand the person well enough to respond productively. To gain the information and insight we require for that understanding, we must listen.

Skill 3: Listen

To actively pursue something is to purposely act to bring it about. To be passive is to sit back and wait to see if it will come to you. To **listen** to someone is to purposely ensure that you have really heard what they are saying. It is you taking responsibility for understanding, rather than making the other person responsible for explaining. To do that you have to really see the individuals in front of you, focus on them, do not allow yourself to be distracted by other things going on around you, or by anything about them—what they are wearing, how they are speaking, or how they look. Give them your full attention and let them know they have it. Look them in the eye (try to get on eye level); unfold your arms; do not fidget; listen to what they are saying. Do not judge what they are saying, do not think about how to reply; focus everything on making sure that you hear and understand. Do not let loose ends dangle. If something does not seem to fit, or if you do not understand what has been said, even if it requires asking personal questions, ask.

Skill 4: Ask

Most people have comfort zones and do not often or easily move beyond their boundaries. Health care professionals cannot afford to allow personal boundaries to limit their ability to provide effective health care; they must be able to do what is necessary. Listening openly without judgment creates the ability to ask direct questions because those questions are being asked in the best interests of the patient. Do not hesitate, simply **ask** for the information and clarification that you need; but do not ask if you do not want to know. There are reasons that people hesitate to be open with each other. Complete candor is often met with criticism or even rejection. If you want others to be open and honest with you, you must be able to accept what they have to say; you must be able to accept them.

Skill 5: Accept

To **accept** another person is to receive them willingly, to respond favorably to them. To reject another person is to refuse to receive them willingly, to refuse to respond favorably to them. In the world around us there is a sea of difference. Age, lifestyle, race, nationality, language, culture, religion, status, appearance, values, ethics, ability, income, education, sexual orientation, interests, politics, and many, many other issues separate us from each other. As adults we work to avoid those separations by constructing a territory containing others who are enough like us for us to understand them. That understanding allows us to make sense of our world and get our needs met. It is easy to care about, accept, and help those who are like us, whom we understand, especially when we see them as needing help through no fault of their own. Whatever has happened to them we can see the possibility of it also happening to us. But what of others whom we do not understand? What of those whose misfortune may seem to us to have been brought about by their own bad, weak, or even immoral choices? We all have our prejudices, which are at the limit of our ability to understand or accept. How do we move past those limitations and receive others willingly, respond favorably to them? The choice may be as simple as yes or no. Creation begins with yes. Stagnation begins with no. Are we trying to create, improve, or encourage something in them? Or are we trying to defend something in us? In which case we will often discourage and destroy something in them. In the end we make a choice. That choice has little to do with the other person standing before us; it is our choice made for our reasons. Will we choose to defend us or to help them? One of the truly remarkable human ironies is that the more we choose ourselves, the less we become, and the more we choose others, the more we are. Accept the human being in front of you. You do not need to understand them. They are the product of their genetics and their world just as you are the product of yours. Relax and continue to do the best you can to take care of what they need.

Skill 6: Encourage

Courage is the will to act in the face of opposition, whether that opposition is from nature, other people, or is found within our own body or mind. That struggle is personal and private, but we are social beings who require the love, acceptance, and respect of others to gain the ability to stand alone. Sometimes all it takes is one person who cares about us and believes in us to give us the courage we need. To encourage someone is to inspire them with courage or hope; to support them in their efforts. Health care professionals, who often enter a person's life at a critical time, can choose to inspire that courage and hope or they can choose to discourage; to deprive others of enthusiasm or courage, to hinder them with disfavor. Each person who influences another's life needs to understand the power for good or ill that they hold. To **encourage**, show confidence in people, build on their strengths; value them, and stimulate their independence. You discourage when you have negative expectations, focus on mistakes, expect perfection, or give too much protection. To help people become more capable, motivate them to believe in themselves and their own abilities. To do that work together with them and demonstrate what you want from them, let them try, acknowledge their efforts, give clear and honest feedback on their performance, refine your demonstration of what you want if necessary, and let them continue to try. For tasks that are difficult for people to accomplish you may need to repeat this process several times, but as they gain new abilities their confidence and independence will grow. Never give up on them and do it yourself. That may take less time initially, and may even seem kind, but it demonstrates your belief that they are not capable; it discourages them and hampers their development.

Skill 7: Assertiveness

Assertiveness is the ability to be aware of what is happening, communicate that awareness, and decide how you will respond to it. When coupled with truly looking at, listening to, accepting, feeling empathy for, and professionally acting in the best interests of the client, this produces a health care provider who can be remarkably insightful and who does not waste much time beating around the bush. This directness is useful in many ways. Following are some suggestions of direct statements or questions that you might use with a client.

For identifying and clarifying client issues:

I have noticed how little you have eaten since you arrived; I wonder how you are feeling about being here.

I hear you when you tell me that you feel well, but I notice that you move very carefully when you go to your right. I wonder if something there is still bothering you.

I see sadness in your eyes; I wonder if you would like to talk about it.

For **anger management**:

Anger is an emotion of last resort intended to drive actions to bring about a change. It can come from any number of different feelings such as feeling threatened, humiliated, frustrated, confused, manipulated, taken advantage of, overwhelmed, inadequate, or inferior, and it is our response when we want the situation to change but don't know what to do to change it. At times like these we do not know what emotions and actions (behaviors) to use so we turn the feeling into the emotion of anger, which drives us to do something even if it is wrong. If we know what to do and are confident in our ability to do it there is no need for anger. If we have no idea of what to do or have no faith in our ability to do it we choose anger. Good interpersonal skills such as really looking at and accepting the person confronting us, waiting to make an appraisal, listening to what he or she is saying, asking for information and understanding we need, and trying to put ourselves in their place, can help to prevent anger most of the time. But these skills need to be combined with assertiveness, because strong feelings are going to drive some sort of behavior, and if we do not choose the behavior ourselves, sooner or later anger will erupt and choose it for us. Following are some statements or questions that may help a client (or you) manage anger.

You seem to me to be purposefully acting in ways and saying things to try to make me angry. Is that true? If so, why would you want to do that?

I know that your mother's accident and her admission here has been a shock to you; please give yourself time to adjust to it all and do not make a decision in anger.

I know that you are angry and feel like lashing out; there is the trash can—kick it. When you have gotten some of it out of your system we will talk.

I am having a hard time being patient with your behavior today; it may be better for us both if we did not see each other until I am more myself.

For good communication skills:

Communication is the art of transferring meaning from one person to another.

Merely transferring words is not the same thing. Never assume that you understand, especially in important issues. The only way for you to be sure that you understand what is being said is to be assertive and ask. Begin with something like, "Are you saying that …" or, "What I hear you saying is …" Then rephrase what you understood them to say in your own words and ask them to confirm or correct it. Continue this process until both of you are satisfied that you fully understand what the client is saying.

Skill 8: Empathy

The ability to put yourself in someone else's place, to imagine what you would feel like if you were in their situation, can create empathy. **Empathy** is a motivation to help someone based on an inner identification with their feelings. The more we have in common with the person and the more we see them as not being responsible for their situation the easier it is for us to identify with, feel empathy for, and be motivated to help them. The more limited our personal experience is the more narrowly we are inclined to define what a person should be, and the less others measure up to our expectations. Our bias creates prejudgments that eliminate empathy and the motivation to help. This can prevent us from actively working in their best interests and leave us merely performing the tasks required by the job of caretaker. Empathy can be considered a skill because we can work to expose ourselves to an array of others in a variety of settings and situations and search for a common bond in order to develop that skill. The naïve sympathy we feel when we are inexperienced and idealistic can never withstand reality and must be replaced with a deeper, more realistic understanding and appreciation of life and for people. Cultivating that understanding and appreciation, that empathy, requires a purposely open mind and willing spirit.

Objectivity

When empathy is combined with professionally acting in the best interests of the client, productive **objectivity** emerges. Objectivity enables the health care provider to act in the best interests of the client, even if the client does not understand or appreciate it. Sometimes a patient who has just had a knee replacement needs to be pushed past a lot of pain to take those first few steps necessary to regain the ability to walk. The difference between independence and permanent disability can be a health care professional who cares enough to simply not take "I can't" for an answer. Sometimes an alcoholic must be faced with hitting the bottom before they are able to confront their need to get sober. The danger is that sympathetic, well-meaning people will bail them out and allow them to sink slowly. Going the same distance down hill is a lot easier if you do it one step at a time than it is if you are looking over the edge of a 30-foot drop. Someone who is missing work and whose job performance is erratic and declining due to alcohol abuse has a better chance of recovery if they are confronted with their well-documented behavior and given the choice of treatment or termination. Appreciation for past performance and sympathy for them and their family may incline an employer to put up with their declining job performance or make ineffectual efforts to warn them and motivate them.

These efforts are very often unproductive as addiction to alcohol leads to biological changes in the brain that result in the use of poor judgment and continued drinking, even when the situation is dangerous or potentially self-destructive. For employees who rely on their jobs the threat of losing them can sometimes get their attention and provide the needed focus when lesser measures have failed (George Washington University, 2008).

Truly helping people can be hard, and sometimes has nothing to do with making them feel good in the moment. They may not even like you when it is all over, but seeing the knee replacement patient playing with his children in the park, or the alcoholic in a restaurant enjoying dinner with his family from the wages of his productive employment, carries a meaning and a satisfaction beyond whether they smile and wave at you.

Skill 9: Behavioral Modification

Behavioral modification is influencing behavior over time. Since behavior is driven by needs, that influence stems from the ability of one person to meet the needs of another (see Figure 6.2).

Our territory is composed of the people, places, and things that we rely on to meet our needs. Behaviors are strategies that are repeated and learned because they succeed at getting our needs met. Problem behavior can emerge either when a dysfunctional territory teaches behavior (violence, coercion, tantrums, manipulation, sulking) that is not appropriate in a functional territory; or when some change within people (dementia, disability), or their territory (divorce, death, migration) creates a situation in which they are unable to get their needs met. When needs are not met they grow increasingly more powerful and drive behaviors that, lacking effective focus, can become increasingly attention-seeking and disruptive. When a need grows powerful enough people can lose control, and their behavior can become harmful or destructive to themselves or others. The purpose of behavioral modification is to reduce and then remove the inappropriate behavior by helping people learn to get their needs met in appropriate ways. To gain an understanding of this process it is helpful to separate behavior into its three elements: the stimulus, the behavior, and the response.

Stimulus: The stimulus is what comes just before the behavior and sets it up. It is provided by the setting the behavior takes place in. It is who, what, when, and where. Who is present, what is happening, when is it happening, and where is it happening? Even though an unmet need may always be present, we do not feel it in the same way all the time. Some settings present the opportunity for the need to be met, and when that opportunity arises the unconscious mind sends a flood of neurotransmitters, creating feelings that drive us to act. Whatever creates the possibility for the need to be met is the stimulus.

Behavior: The behavior is the set of emotions and actions that flow from the feeling. It is the effort expended in the attempt to get the need met. Behaviors are learned over time, and specific types of behaviors are used almost automatically to respond to specific types of stimuli. Once a set of behaviors has been formed and linked to a specific stimulus the coupling resists change because it is locked into a physical structure in the brain. New behaviors can be formed and linked to the old stimulus, but it takes time.

Response: The response is the reaction of some element in the territory to the behavior. It is what the person is gaining from it. Most behaviors are learned in childhood because the response of others either meets the child's needs or it does not. Most problem behavior is social behavior intended to gain a reaction from another person. For that reason there is a strong attention-getting component. Attention is looking at, touching, talking to, listening to, or focusing your activity around another person, and most often negative behavior succeeds in gaining a response.

Creating a Behavioral Modification Plan

1. Observe and record.

   - Stimulus: Carefully record who is present; what is happening; when (year, month, week, day, hour, minute); and where a behavior takes place. Look for patterns that would allow you to predict it.

   - Behavior: Exactly what does the person do that presents a problem? How often does the negative behavior happen (frequency), and how long does each episode last (duration)? A record of all of this will become the baseline information that will later allow you to evaluate whether a plan is working.

   - Response: What do other people do when the problem behavior emerges? What is the person getting out of the problem behavior? Most often they will be getting attention; that is, they are being looked at, touched, talked to, listened to, or are controlling the activity of others. You may also find that they are able to get something they want, or avoid something they do not want.

2. Understand what you are trying to do.
   In order to permanently change a behavior you need to stop the negative behavior while you start a positive one. Before making a plan, think through each element of the behavior carefully.

   - Stimulus: Once you have identified the dynamics of the stimulus, how would you avoid them in order to reduce the problem behavior? Confronting a problem behavior while it is happening is a losing proposition. The behavior is being driven by intense feelings and people are generally not capable of being objective at that moment. Confronting people while they are performing a behavior they cannot themselves understand or control can result in hopelessness, or in defensiveness, or even defiance that creates a strong resistance to change. In addition, it is impossible to confront a negative behavior without paying attention to the person for it. Paying attention to negative behavior only encourages and prolongs it.

- Behavior: The behavior is the least important part of the process. It is merely what the person has learned to do in any given situation to get the desired response from others. If the behavior does not succeed in getting that response it will in time be abandoned if another successful behavior can be found. You must teach the person a positive behavior they can perform that will get their needs met. Look for a positive behavior that cannot be performed at the same time as the negative behavior. If the negative behavior is being loud and disruptive to gain attention or get what they want, the positive behavior may be asking for it in a normal tone. Understand that the person will most likely not be able to perform the entire positive behavior well in the beginning, so mold the behavior by at first responding positively to anything that is close to it and then gradually requiring more before you respond. For example, if you want the person to ask for something in a normal tone of voice instead of crying and screaming, you may at first ignore the crying and screaming until he or she becomes silent for a moment and then respond to the silence with attention. Gradually you can decrease the attention given and require the person to be silent for a longer period of time before giving him or her what they want, while you listen for anything said in a normal tone. Each time something is said in a normal tone increase your attention to it, and then reinforce the behavior by paying more attention when the person asks for what they want in that same tone.

- Response: Whatever it is the person is getting out of the negative behavior, you must prevent them from getting it; you have to stop the behavior from working. As long as it works there is no reason for the person to stop using it. However, not allowing a negative behavior to work is not enough. When you prevent a behavior from working you stop people from getting their needs met, and those needs will grow to drive ever more disruptive behaviors. Things almost always get worse before they get better. As the need grows stronger people have to discover that they are able to meet that need by using a different behavior. In order for them to make that discovery you must begin responding in a positive way to the behavior you want. That positive response needs to come from inside of you, and it needs to be genuine. The more you care and the better connection you make with the person whose behavior you are trying to change, the better it will work. Rewards can never replace caring. The use of rewards given for positive behavior is helpful if the person needs a physical symbol of your approval, appreciation, and respect for his or her effort, but it is your genuine positive response that motivates the change, not the reward. The needs you are trying to meet are the needs for safety and security, love, acceptance and belonging, respect, and self-respect. The only way people will know that they have any of those things is by seeing it in your response to them. When you respond to their behavior with those qualities, people will strive to duplicate the behavior. Remember that behavior is complex; it combines an internal state, an emotion, and an external action, and people will not be very good at the new behavior at first. In time, if the negative behavior continues to be unsuccessful and the positive behavior continues to work they will practice the new behavior until they get better at it. The old negative behavior will decline and the new positive behavior will grow.

3. Create the plan.

- Stimulus: What happens that starts the behavior? How will you avoid that situation? Who needs to be included in the plan?

- Behavior: What is the negative behavior that needs to be stopped? What is the positive behavior that needs to be started? If the new behavior is to be molded, what are the steps in the process? Observe to see if the positive behavior is now happening spontaneously. If so, record how often the positive behavior occurs and how long each episode lasts. This will be the baseline data for the positive behavior.

- Response: How will you ignore the negative behavior? How will you attend to the positive behavior? Will the positive behavior need to be molded? If so, what behavior will you attend to in the beginning and how will you help the client to progress to the desired behavior? How will you keep records of how often the negative and positive behaviors take place? How long will you try the plan before evaluating the results to see if it is working?

4. Carry out the plan.

Allow the plan to run for the determined length of time. Do not evaluate it along the way and second-guess it; things will often get worse before they get better. It generally takes three to four weeks to see if it is working or not. Be sure to record how often both negative and positive behaviors occur and how long each episode of negative or positive behavior lasts.

5. Evaluate the results.

At the designated time, compare how often the negative behavior is occurring now with how often it occurred in the baseline data. Also compare how long each episode of problem behavior lasts with how long they lasted in the baseline data. Is the negative behavior happening less often, the same amount, or more often? Is the average length of the negative episodes getting shorter, staying the same, or getting longer? Following are some suggestions for evaluating outcomes of the behavior modification plan.

A. The negative behavior has decreased, or the episodes of negative behavior have decreased in length.
   (i) The plan may be working. Let it run for another two to three weeks and then reevaluate it.
      (a) If the positive behavior has also increased, keep doing what you are doing.
      (b) If the positive behavior has not increased, try molding it (see the example under number 2 above).

B. The negative behavior has increased, or the episodes of negative behavior have increased in length.
   (i) It is likely that you have been successful at not allowing the negative behavior to work. This has caused the need to grow and it is driving increased negative behavior. In addition, it is likely that you have not been able to relieve this need by responding to positive behavior. Check to see if the positive behavior has increased in frequency or duration.
      (a) If the positive behavior has not increased you may need to mold it, that is, look for a simpler part of the behavior that you can attend to (see the example in number 2 above). It is imperative that you deliver attention and relieve the need or it will grow uncontrollable. It is also imperative that this attention be delivered in response to a behavior that at least takes you in the direction of the desired positive behavior. Pick a slightly positive or at least neutral behavior to attend to and start again.

C. Both the positive and the negative behaviors have increased.
   (i) Slightly increase the attention you are giving to the positive behavior and be sure that the negative behavior is not allowed to work, and that as little attention is paid to it as possible. The negative behavior will struggle on for a while, but it will decrease in time. Let the program run for two to three more weeks and then reevaluate.

D. There has been no significant change in the positive or in the negative behavior.
   (i) The person or people delivering the attention may not matter to the one whose behavior they are trying to change. The reason for social behavior is to get a response from others who are in a position to meet our needs.

There are people with whom we have a connection and whose positive regard and respect matter very much to us, and there are people with whom we have no connection and whose positive regard and respect matter very little to us. The greater the connection we have with someone, the more influence he or she has on our behavior. If the connection is great enough, no behavioral plan is necessary; just that person's positive expectation of us is enough to change our behavior. If you want to influence people's behavior really look at them, do not rush to judgment, actively listen to them, ask them openly about things you do not understand about them, accept them, encourage them, care enough to work for their best interests, and always, always respect them. Make that connection and you will have more effect on their life than the greatest behavioral technician on earth could ever imagine.

Special Circumstances

In situations that prevent people from appropriately planning or carrying out behaviors, they cease to be able to get their needs met. Mental illness or dementia (see Chapter 9) prevent a person from mentally processing a setting accurately, and produce behavior that others do not understand or respond well to. People with mental illness or dementia are unable to take effective action to meet their needs, which then grow and produce powerful feelings that may turn outward and drive disruptive attention-getting behaviors, or turn inward and collapse into depression and despair. Whether a person is unintelligible and disruptive or distant and nonresponsive, their needs do not change. Everyone needs the same things: safety and security, love, acceptance and belonging, respect, and self-respect. When a person loses the ability to provide for their own needs it becomes the responsibility of others, especially health care professionals, to make provisions for them. The elderly resident of a nursing home who lives with dementia needs to feel physically comfortable, safe and secure, to love and be loved; to care for and be cared for, to feel needed and to be useful, and to feel good about themselves—but they have lost the ability to understand what is happening to them or to communicate their needs to others. Because of this, when these needs emerge and grow strong they may communicate them by screaming, crying for help, or with anger or hostility. These actions may seem to make no sense to an observer, but they do make sense from the perspective of a person with dementia. The internal experiences and what it takes to meet the needs of each dementia patient are unique, but discovering and providing for those needs will reduce or eliminate the behaviors by making them unnecessary. For a discussion on the practice of dementia care that is beyond the scope of this book read *The Art of Dementia Care* by Daniel Kuhn and Jane Verity published by Cengage/Delmar Learning.

SUMMARY

Humankind has a long history of caring for those who cannot care for themselves. In part this is due to the fact that we are social beings drawn to each other and kept together by needs that only others can fill. In order to be functional and stable the social relationships that emerge as we are drawn together must meet the needs of all of the individuals involved. If a relationship does not meet the needs of one or more of the individuals those needs will grow and strain the relationship, as they focus those people on themselves and drive self-centered behaviors designed to get those needs met. Those self-serving behaviors do not if a person is supposed to be caring for someone else. Even a professional relationship, which exists to provide for the needs of the client, most often meets some of the social needs of the provider. Our needs to belong, to be respected and to respect ourselves (esteem), and our need for self-actualization can all be met by supervisors, peers, or by the clients or patients themselves. Whether or not our needs are being met can depend as much on what we need as on how others respond to us. The lowest-order need that is chronically unmet grows until it dominates the individual and motivates behavior at that level. Moral levels are defined by why we do what we do, by our motivation; and there is a characteristic moral level for each need level. The higher the level of need that is motivating us the less we require a positive response from others to meet that need. Also the better our needs are being met in our personal relationships the less we depend on positive responses in our professional relationships. Healthy personal development and satisfying personal relationships are some of our most powerful professional assets.

Skills are learned abilities that increase our ability to care for others. Really looking at and seeing others, not rushing to judgment, actively listening, openly asking to understand, accepting others, encouragement, assertiveness, anger management, empathy, objectivity, and behavioral modification are all abilities that improve with practice and that increase our ability to understand, withstand, respond appropriately to, and motivate others.

APPLICATION SKILL

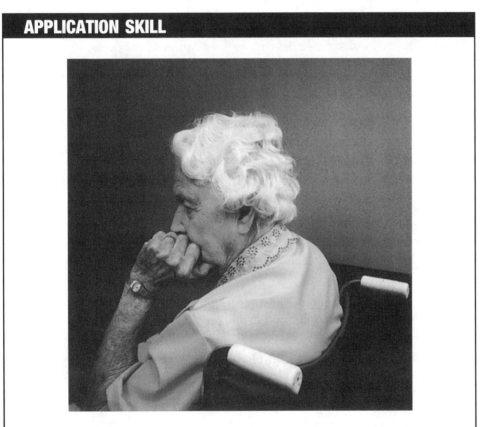

Encourage

To encourage is to inspire someone with courage or hope; to support them.

Humankind is an enigma; each of us is a social being who requires the love, acceptance, and respect of others in order to gain the ability to stand alone. Courage is the will to act in the face of opposition, whether that opposition is from nature, other people, or is found within our own body or mind. Sometimes all it takes is one person who cares about us and believes in us to give us the courage we need.

The 78-year-old nursing home resident has the flu and she is shutting-down and dying. She has been a resident for just over a year and her family, who live a distance away, have stopped visiting on a regular basis. She is aware that she will never be able to live independently and she feels like a burden. You are powerless to change the reality of her situation. How do you encourage her?

APPLICATION SKILL (continued)

Life is lived in moments. You have already helped by the positive attention you are giving. When we dwell on what we do not have we tend to forget what we do have. Help her talk about the simple things she enjoys in life—her favorite television program, donuts on Friday mornings, playing Bingo with her friends. Find a way to make her laugh. Then get on the phone and get her family to visit her and let her know they care.

Health care professionals, family, friends, teachers, supervisors, and, more often than you would think, complete strangers, are in a position to inspire courage in others; or they can choose to discourage them and deprive them of enthusiasm or courage, hinder them by disfavoring. Each person who influences someone else's life needs to understand the power for good or ill that they hold.

To encourage, show confidence in people, build on their strengths, value them, and stimulate their independence. You discourage when you have negative expectations, focus on mistakes, expect perfection, or give too much protection. To help people become more capable, motivate them to believe in themselves and their abilities. To do that, work together with them and demonstrate what you want from them, let them try, acknowledge their efforts, give clear and honest feedback on their performance, refine your demonstration of what you want if necessary, and let them continue to try. For tasks that are difficult for them you may need to repeat this process several times, but as people gain new abilities their confidence and independence will grow. Never give up on them and do it yourself. That may take less time initially, and may even seem kind, but it demonstrates your belief that they are not capable; it discourages them and hampers their development.

CONCEPT REVIEW

history of caring – Humankind has a long history of caring for those in need. Early modern human and Neanderthal burials excavated from over 100,000 years ago reveal healed areas on bones that would have been devastating breaks and that would have required the care and support of others for the individual to have survived long enough to heal.

social beings – Humans are social beings; many needs can only be met through relationships with others.

moral levels – Moral levels are defined not by what we do, but by why we do it. As the lowest order need that is chronically unmet grows powerful it motivates behavior that can most often be defined and predicted by the morals at that level.

needs correlated with moral levels – (a) physical needs: power; (b) safety and security needs: deals; (c) love needs: good boy/good girl; (d) belonging needs: rules (authority); (e) esteem needs: social contracts; (f) self-actualization needs: individual conscience.

altruism – The willingness to sacrifice your own good for the benefit of another. Individuals who score high on the personality trait of agreeableness are genuinely concerned for the welfare of others and are more likely to be altruistic.

skills – Providing care for others involves behaviors that must be learned. Each health care specialty has its own specific skill set, but there are also skill areas that are helpful in every specialty because they are helpful in dealing with people, and with the stresses involved.

look – The primary method of gathering information about others; it utilizes an extensive development in the brain devoted to gathering and interpreting non-verbal information.

wait – Avoiding the natural impulse to make snap judgments of others and taking the time needed to form a broader, more realistic appraisal.

listen – Active listening is purposely engaging in the process of listening to ensure that you have really heard and understood what the other person is saying.

ask – Moving beyond the normal boundaries of conversation and assertively asking for the information and clarification you need to understand the patient.

accept – To receive another willingly, to respond favorably to them.

encouragement – Defined in Webster's Collegiate Dictionary as "to inspire with courage or hope; to support."

assertiveness – The ability to be aware of what is happening, to communicate that awareness, and decide how you will respond to it.

anger Management – The development of skills to avoid or redirect anger to prevent it from driving unproductive or self-destructive behavior.

communication – The art of accurately transferring meaning from one person to another.

empathy – A motivation to help other people based on an inner identification with their feelings. Empathy can be created by the ability to mentally put yourself in their place, to feel what it would be like if you were in their situation.

objectivity – Empathy combined with professional behavior toward the client produces the ability to act in the best interests of the client, even if the client does not understand or appreciate it.

behavioral modification – Influencing behavior over time.

stimulus – What comes just before the behavior and sets it up. It is provided by the setting the behavior takes place in. It is who, what, when, and where.

behavior – The set of emotions and actions that flow from feelings. It is the effort expended in the attempt to meet a need.

response – The reaction of some element in the territory to a behavior. It is what the person gains from the behavior. If a behavior is successful, the response meets the need that drove the behavior.

REVIEW QUESTIONS

I.   Completion

Complete the following sentences.

1. Sacrificing yourself for the good of another is
   _____.

2. A relationship that exists for the good of the client, and for which a provider receives payment is a _____ relationship.

3. Acting in the best interests of the client, even if the client does not understand or appreciate it is _____.

4. _____ are defined by our motivations, by why we do something rather than by what we do.

5. The ability to put yourself in someone else's shoes, to see things from their perspective and identify with their feelings, is
   _____.

II.   Multiple Choice

Select the letter of the choice that best completes the statement.

6. A relationship that exists only to meet the needs of one person may be (circle all that apply)
   A. Dysfunctional
   B. Functional
   C. Professional
   D. Social

7. Helping someone to find hope and motivation is
   A. Assertiveness
   B. Encouragement
   C. Active listening
   D. Communication

8. Ensuring that you understand the full meaning of what someone else is saying is
   A. Assertiveness
   B. Encouragement
   C. Active listening
   D. Communication

9. Remaining in control of your emotions while under attack and staying focused on the issue at hand best describes:
   A. Assertiveness
   B. Professionalism
   C. Non-defensiveness
   D. Anger management

10. The ability to be aware of what is happening, communicate that awareness, and decide how you will respond to it.
    A. Assertiveness
    B. Professionalism
    C. Non-defensiveness
    D. Anger management

III.   Matching

Match each term with its correct description.

    A. Individual conscience
    B. Deals
    C. Rules
    D. Good boy/good girl
    E. Power
    F. Social contracts

_____ Motivation for behavior designed to respond to chronically unmet physical needs.

_____ Motivation for behavior designed to meet chronically unmet belonging needs.

_____ Motivation for behavior designed to meet chronically unmet needs for love.

_____ Motivation for behavior designed to meet chronically unmet needs to be safe and secure.

IV.   Critical Thinking

11. Explain your answer(s) to question number six.

12. Give one advantage and one disadvantage of waiting to gain information and insight before making an appraisal of someone.

13. How can your sympathy for another help them? How can it hurt them?

14. Why do you think people risk their lives to help strangers?

15. How can being unable to meet your own needs limit your ability to help someone else?

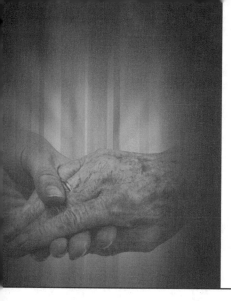

Chapter 7

Upon completion of this chapter you should be able to:

1. Define a professional relationship.
2. Define and list examples of helping relationships.
3. Define and discuss the need for financial boundaries.
4. Define and discuss the need for physical boundaries.
5. Define and discuss the need for emotional boundaries.
6. State the area of the professional relationship regulated by the federal government.
7. State the area of the professional relationship regulated by the state government.
8. Discuss the purpose and effect of case law.
9. Define and discuss the need for informed consent.
10. Discuss the practice of common courtesy.
11. Define and discuss the need for privacy.
12. Define and discuss the need for confidentiality.
13. Define and discuss the implications of beneficence.
14. Define and discuss the implications of nonmaleficence.
15. Define and discuss the implications of physician-centered medical care and identify its contribution to current medical practice.
16. Define and discuss the implications of client-centered medical care and identify its contribution to current medical practice.
17. Identify reasons for the development of payment-centered medical care.
18. Define and discuss the implications of payment-centered medical care.
19. Define patient advocacy and discuss its contribution to current medical practice.
20. Describe issues needing to be addressed for effective health care reform and contrast these with the current practice of medical care.

KEY TERMS

professional	state regulation	nonmaleficence
professional relationship	case law	doctor-centered
helping relationship	informed consent	client-centered
financial boundaries	courtesy	payment-centered
physical boundaries	privacy	health care reform
emotional boundaries	confidentiality	
federal regulation	beneficence	

The Professional Medical Relationship

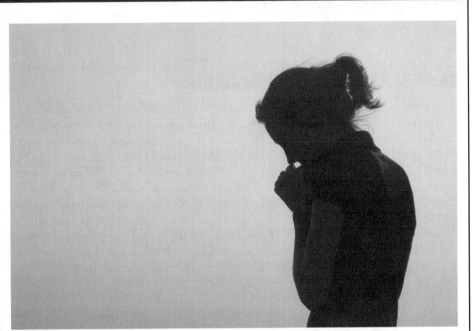

Assertiveness

You have recently taken your first job as a technician in a hospital psychiatric ward and on this shift for the first time have been assigned to the geriatric unit. During your shift you observe other technicians ignoring the direction of the charge nurse and doing very little to provide care for their charges. When they do engage patients some of them even generate conflict with the patients, during which they humiliate and hurt them. The charge nurse is aware of what is happening and when you question her, she turns away from you without reply. When you address the other technicians they describe a litany of patient hostility and misbehavior, showing you fresh bruises and healed scars incurred during the performance of their duties. They explain that the patients know exactly what they are doing and can control their own behavior if they want, so are being hurtful and hostile on purpose and therefore deserve everything they get. The technicians go on to claim that the way they treat the patients is the only thing that keeps them under control and that should they stop treating them as they do, the patients will very quickly harm themselves and each other. As they finish you notice a circle of experienced technicians and nurses watching you and waiting for your reaction. You really need this job. What do you do?

INTRODUCTION

This chapter is about the nature of a professional relationship and the boundaries, regulatory bodies, and ethics involved in professional relationships in the health care industry. These define, encompass, and ensure patient rights and provider responsibilities and have developed over the years guided by three distinct philosophies that have governed medical practice at different times. Pressure is growing for health care reform to develop a new, fourth philosophy to govern current and future medical practice.

Look for the definition of professional relationships; the physical, emotional, and financial boundaries that ensure them; and the areas of regulation supplied by the federal and state governments and by the courts. Also look for the patient's rights of informed consent, privacy, and confidentiality and the provider's responsibilities of beneficence and nonmaleficence—the three philosophies that have contributed to the development of those rights and responsibilities as they governed health care through the years; the current state of the health care industry; and the requirements of effective health care reform.

After studying this section you should have a clearer understanding of the nature of a professional relationship in the health care industry; why it exists, how it developed, how it is protected and enforced, its current state, and the direction that reform needs to take.

THE PROFESSIONAL RELATIONSHIP

A **professional** is someone who is skilled and who is paid to apply that skill. When the skill involves a service to another person, the professional is paid to use their skill to perform the service for the good of the client and a **professional relationship** is understood to exist. This is not an entirely new kind of relationship. It is only an extreme example of what this book refers to as a helping relationship. A **helping relationship** is one in which one person takes the responsibility for doing what is in the best interests of another. Helping relationships can include parent–child relations, friendship, teaching, mentoring, nursing, aid, and many other such endeavors, as long as one is truly acting in the best interests of the other. There was a time when one person could do most of these things for another, but as society became more complex, at some point the skill needed to help in more than one specific way became too great for one person, and people began to specialize. As the time necessary to develop and employ a necessary skill increased, a specialist did not have the time to devote to earning his or her own livelihood by traditional means, and required payment from those being helped. Nevertheless, the point of the relationship was not the payment made, it was the help needed. Professional relationships today continue this tradition. The profession exists for the needs of the client.

Professional Boundaries

As we saw in Chapter 6, professionals are as human as anyone, and if their needs are not met their ability to meet their client's needs may be jeopardized; but this has nothing to do with the client. Professionals are responsible for their own needs and for the level of care they provide. In order to keep this all in a clear perspective, a professional relationship contains very specific financial, physical, and emotional boundaries.

- **Financial boundaries** involve payment.   Professionals are paid to apply their skill. Without payment a professional relationship does not exist. Hospitals, nursing homes, doctors, laboratories, and clinics are all careful to make arrangements for payment prior to the delivery of services.

- **Physical boundaries** regard touch.   As much as it is possible, touch a client only with their permission and always touch only when it is appropriate. Respect the client's personal space. Sexual contact and harsh or punitive contact is never appropriate. Touch can be an important part of a helping relationship, but always be aware of how the client is responding. Touch can easily be misinterpreted as too personal.

- **Emotional boundaries** involve objectivity. Compassion and care cannot be allowed to cloud your professional judgment. The sympathetic nurse who does not push the knee replacement patient into trying to use his new knee and putting weight on it has become part of the problem, not the solution. Sending a lonely and homesick patient home before they are physically ready may seem like kindness until they fall and hemorrhage at home. There is a reason that professionals do not provide services to those closest to them; when emotional attachment overrides professional judgment there is too great a chance of harm, rather than help, being the outcome.

Regulation

Health care professions are regulated at three levels: the federal government, the state governments, and the courts.

- **Federal regulation.** The highest level of legal control is at the level of the federal government. Federal legislation regulates third party payees. There are two parties to a professional relationship, the provider and the client. If someone else is paying for it they are known as the third party payee. Federal legislation covers insurance companies, health maintenance organizations, Medicaid, and Medicare.
- **State regulation.** The next level of control is invested in each state government. Each state regulates the actual practice of medicine with Professional Practices Acts that govern the activities of hospitals, nursing homes, Medicaid programs, and medical professionals within that state.
- Courts. Legal interpretations of medical regulations are established by **case law** as medical questions are brought before the court. New law can be established with each case, although every judge is bound by the decisions made by all judges before them. Case law can only be overturned by the state or federal Supreme Court.

Medical Ethics

Medical ethics are rules that regulate the practice of medicine with regard to patient rights and provider responsibilities.

- Patient's rights. The rights of the client are based on the concept of autonomy, the right to self-determination, and are protected by the practice of informed consent.
- **Informed consent.** Clients have the right to be informed of their diagnosis in a language they understand, what treatment is being proposed, the possible risks and benefits of the proposed treatment and of non-treatment, and of reasonable alternatives to the proposed treatment. Clients must sign a statement indicating that these things have been explained to them, that they understand them, and that they accept the proposed treatment.
- **Courtesy.** Clients have the right to be treated with courtesy and respect. Harsh, demeaning, or harassing actions or words by health care providers are never appropriate.
- **Privacy.** Clients have the right to privacy. Some necessary conversations and procedures may invade the client's privacy, but these are always performed with the client's knowledge and permission and always in as private a setting as possible; people not directly involved or necessary to the procedure should not be there without the expressed approval of the client.
- **Confidentiality.** Clients have the right to confidentiality. Anything you learn about the client is given to you in trust, and information about a client, either medical or personal—even the fact that the client is at your facility—can never be shared without the client's written permission.

Provider Responsibilities

The responsibilities of the provider include beneficence and nonmaleficence.

- **Beneficence.**   Do good; all that is done should be done for the good of the patient. This is the central issue of the professional relationship itself. The relationship exists only for the good of the client. The case study at the beginning of this chapter clearly illustrates the devastating effects that violation of this precept can have on the patient.

- **Nonmaleficence.**   Do no harm; the benefit of treatment must clearly outweigh the risk of harm. Experimental treatment is only appropriate with the client's full knowledge and approval, and surgery or other invasive procedures that are unnecessary are never appropriate. This leads to the question of who decides what is necessary and what is unnecessary. The answer to that has changed over the years.

HISTORY OF HEALTH CARE

There have been three distinct philosophies that have governed the provision of health care through the years. These might be characterized as the doctor-centered, client-centered, and payment-centered phases.

- **Doctor-centered** phase.   Until the 1960s, doctors were seen as the experts and most people followed their directions without question (Cassell, 2000). This was a "father knows best" style of medicine. It was based on the good of the client but not their rights. Information was often withheld, treatments could be forced, and involuntary commitment was relatively simple, all based solely on the doctor's evaluation. The civil rights movement of the 1960s led to a new philosophy, the client-centered approach, in which the client's rights became more central.

- **Client-centered** phase.   Growing from the civil rights movement of the 1960s, this phase placed the client at the center: the doctor was seen as a consultant who provided information and advice, but the patient made the decisions (Siegler, 2000). The patient became a client who could shop around, consulting different doctors until they got an answer they liked. Using this approach, clients became much more active in the health care process, but there was pressure on doctors to provide answers that clients liked, and what clients wanted was not always what they needed. Regardless of who was making the decisions, doctors were still liable for their advice. Lawsuits for malpractice grew out of control and many providers began to practice "defensive medicine" (Sulmasy, 1997), suggesting every conceivable diagnostic procedure and recommending the most aggressive treatments.

- **Payment-centered** phase.   Beginning in the 1980s the concern for client's rights, the high cost of malpractice suits, and rapid advances in medicine—leading to rapid advances in medical costs (Loewy, 1987)—led to the development of complex regulatory codes, client's rights laws, strict adherence to medical protocol to avoid lawsuits, and insurance payment limitations to contain costs. This pushed the practice of medicine to ignore individual needs or responses in favor of "by the book" practices that were only partially based on the good of the client (Minogue, 2000).

    Every new innovation of medical science is wonderful for the diagnosis or treatment of the patient, but can require the purchase of terribly expensive machinery and the employment of highly skilled technicians, both of which raise the cost of medical care. And medical science is innovating and discovering at a record pace. Hospitals that used to be able to afford to provide a wide range of free services to people who could not afford them have to limit those services or be faced with going bankrupt, and one after another small, independent hospitals and clinics have been forced to sell themselves to larger chains that are able to modernize. But modernizing also means economizing: cutting staff, limiting free services, and using less qualified (less expensive) personnel for many functions. Health care providers are now accountable to government agencies, hospitals, and insurance companies as well as their clients. The good of the client has been largely replaced by the need of the health care system to contain costs as the first priority. It does no good to offer phenomenal services for two years and then have to close the hospital and serve no one. More people receive more care in the long run if you keep the system viable. But there are always those who limit services simply to maintain high profits.

HEALTH CARE ADVOCATES

In this confusing health care climate, patients must be very capable of advocating for themselves or they must have someone who is strong and well-acquainted with the system helping them if they are to get the best care possible. Both services and care have become limited, and if someone is not strongly advocating for them clients are at risk of receiving an unacceptable level of treatment and care (Drench et al., 2003).

Limitations of services due to reductions of insurance coverage and the necessity of spending large amounts of already limited time justifying the need for any treatment not on the insurance company's approved list can lead doctors to not recommend some procedures. Only someone well-acquainted with the health care system would even be aware of the need to question that. One possible future for health care is the expansion of the number of specialist nurses who work for the patient to ensure due diligence in diagnosis and treatment, and in nursing care.

The need for such specialization is also driven by the downsizing of nursing staff that has left fewer health care workers caring for patients. This can leave patients vying for the attention of care providers, and as those providers scramble to keep up it is all too easy to pass the quiet patient by and deliver services to the one who is more vocal, even if the quieter patient needs it more. Sometimes care providers end a shift feeling as though they have spent their time putting out fires and are all too aware of the things they could not get done, all of the care they could not deliver.

HEALTH CARE REFORM

The issues listed above assume that the person is receiving medical care. Despite the truly admirable efforts of a range of free and sliding-scale clinics and services donated by hospitals, millions of people in the United States are uninsured or underinsured and are unable to access or afford care. Ironically, this allows small health issues to grow into large ones before care can be accessed, turning small costs into large, at times enormous, costs for the health care system. Health insurance that could prevent this escalation is simply too expensive for most individuals to afford. Small businesses often struggle with the high cost of premiums for their employees, if they are able to afford them at all, with the largest companies paying the lowest per person premiums. Even with health insurance, coverage for long-term care is almost unheard of. **Health care reform** is needed that balances individual freedom with public good; achieves cost containment through community-based public health prevention programs that remove the causes of disease and provide early diagnosis and treatment to prevent small disorders from growing into large problems; and provides acceptable levels of care and equal access to all, including long-term care. Whether health care remains in the private sector or comes under the public domain will likely be determined by whether or not the private sector carries out such reform on its own before sufficient voter emotion is aroused to activate government control. Any way we go there are some hard choices to make. How do we balance individual freedom with the reality of health care dollars? Do we continue to allow individuals the right to choose high-risk activities such as smoking? If we do, we will continue to pay for it with the much larger share of the health care budget that the effects of those activities require. How much of the national budget are we willing to devote to health care? If we spend more, do we raise taxes to pay for it? Or do we cut back on other federal services? How much money do we spend trying to save a person with a 5 percent chance of survival? Does it matter if that person is one month old or ninety years old? If it costs a million dollars to treat someone with a 90 percent chance of survival is the cost too high? There are only so many health care dollars to go around, and we have to ask how many others could be saved with the money we are spending on any one person. Are some lives worth more than others so that we will spend more on saving them? Is it fair to save one person at the expense of losing five? Sometimes if you save one person's leg you lose another person's life. The day may be coming when the rights and even the good of the individual will have to be balanced with the needs of the society.

SUMMARY

A professional is someone who is skilled and who is paid to apply that skill for the benefit of another. The professional relationship is only one of many types of helping relationships in which one person takes the responsibility for doing what is in the best interests of another. In order to ensure that a professional relationship exists there are very specific financial, physical, and emotional boundaries, and health care professions are regulated at three levels: by the federal government, by the state governments, and by the courts.

Medical ethics are rules that regulate the practice of medicine with regard to the patient's rights to informed consent, privacy, and confidentiality, as well as the provider's responsibilities of beneficence and nonmaleficence (to work in the best interests of and to not harm the client). These rights and responsibilities have been shaped by three distinct philosophies that have governed the provision of health care through the years. These might be characterized as the doctor-centered, client-centered, and payment-centered phases. In the payment-centered philosophy as it exists today, both services and care have been limited to reduce costs, and if someone is not strongly advocating for them clients may be at risk of receiving an unacceptable level of treatment and care. The health care system in the United States is out of balance, and health care reform is needed that achieves cost containment through public health, prevention programs, and early diagnosis and treatment, and that provides acceptable levels of care and equal access to all, including long-term care.

APPLICATION SKILL

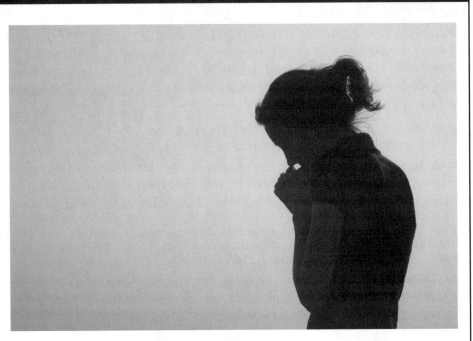

Assertiveness

You have recently taken your first job as a technician in a hospital psychiatric ward and on this shift have been assigned to the geriatric unit for the first time. During your shift you observe other technicians ignoring the direction of the charge nurse and doing very little to provide care for their charges. When they do engage patients some of them even generate conflict with the patients, during which they humiliate and hurt them. The charge nurse is aware of what is happening and when you question her she turns away from you without reply. When you address the other technicians they describe a litany of patient hostility and misbehavior, showing you fresh bruises and healed scars incurred in the performance of their duties. They explain that the patients know exactly what they are doing and can control their own behavior if they want, so are being hurtful and hostile on purpose and therefore deserve everything they get. They go on to claim that the way they treat the patients is the only thing that keeps them under control and that should they stop treating them as they do the patients will very quickly harm themselves and each other. As they finish you notice a circle of experienced technicians and nurses watching you and waiting for your reaction. You really need this job. What do you do?

The professional relationship leaves no room for debate regarding this decision. The reason that you and the rest of the staff are employed here is for the good of the patients, who are being humiliated and hurt. What you have seen and heard must be reported to the management of the hospital and to the appropriate agency for the aging in your state. No one ever comes away from a battle without scars and you will take several hits in this one. Any reasonable person would desire to avoid the conflict if possible, but there is a time when a person must take a stand, even if they stand alone. Assertiveness is the ability to be aware of what is happening, communicate that awareness, and decide how you will respond to it. When combined with truly looking at, listening to, accepting, feeling empathy for, and professionally acting in the best interests of the client, a health care provider emerges who can be remarkably insightful and who does not waste much time beating around the bush. Following is a suggestion for assertively responding to the above situation:

I hear what you are saying and think that you may even believe that it is true, but it seems to me that you have lost the meaning of why we are here. I will have to report what I have seen to all of the appropriate places.

(See Appendix A for state hot-line numbers.)

See Chapter 6 for additional examples of assertive statements.

CONCEPT REVIEW

professional – Someone who is skilled and who is paid to apply that skill for the benefit of another.

professional relationship – Exists when the professional is paid to perform their skill as a personal service for the benefit of another person.

helping relationship – A relationship in which one person takes the responsibility for doing what is in the best interests of another.

financial boundaries – Involve payment. Professionals are paid to apply their skill. Without payment a professional relationship does not exist.

physical boundaries – Regard touch. As much as is possible touch a client only with their permission and always touch only when it is appropriate.

emotional boundaries – Involve objectivity. Compassion and care cannot be allowed to cloud professional judgment.

federal regulations – Govern third party payees such as insurance companies, health maintenance organizations, Medicaid, and Medicare.

state regulations – Govern the actual practice of medicine with professional practices acts that apply to the activities of hospitals, nursing homes, Medicaid programs, and medical professionals within the state.

case law – Established by legal interpretations of medical regulations as medical questions are brought before the court. New law can be established with each case, as every judge is bound by the decisions made by all judges before them. Case Law can only be overturned by the state or federal Supreme Court.

medical ethics – Rules that regulate the practice of medicine with regard to patient rights and provider responsibilities.

patient's rights – Based on the concept of autonomy, the right to self-determination, and are protected by the practice of informed consent.

informed consent – Clients have the right to be informed of their diagnosis in a language they understand, what treatment is being proposed, the possible risks and benefits of the proposed treatment and of non-treatment, and reasonable alternatives to the proposed treatment. Clients must sign a statement indicating that these things have been explained to them, that they understand them, and that they accept the proposed treatment.

courtesy – Clients have the right to be treated with courtesy and respect. Harsh, demeaning, or harassing actions or words by health care providers are never appropriate.

privacy – Clients have the right to privacy. Some necessary conversations and procedures invade the client's privacy, but these are always performed with the client's knowledge and permission and always in as private a setting as possible. People not directly involved in and necessary to the procedure should not be there without the expressed approval of the client.

confidentiality – Clients have the right to confidentiality. Anything you learn about the client is given to you in trust, and information about a client, either medical or personal, even the fact that the client is at your facility, can never be shared without the client's written permission.

provider responsibilities – The responsibilities of the provider include beneficence and nonmaleficence.

beneficence – Do good; all that is done should be done for the good of the patient.

nonmaleficence – Do no harm; the benefit of treatment must clearly outweigh the risk of harm.

history of health care – There have been three distinct philosophies that have governed the provision of health care through the years. These might be characterized as the doctor-centered, client-centered, and payment-centered phases.

doctor-centered medical care – Until the 1960s, doctors were seen as the experts and most people followed their directions without question. This was based on the good of the client but not their rights. Information was often withheld, treatments could be forced, and involuntary commitment was relatively simple, all based solely on the doctor's evaluation.

client-centered medical care – With the client as the center, the doctor was seen as a consultant who would provide information and advice, but the patient made the decisions. The patient became a client who could shop around, consulting different doctors until they got an answer they liked.

defensive medicine – The response of many doctors to the increased number of lawsuits that resulted from client-centered medical care, defensive medicine involves suggesting every conceivable diagnostic procedure and recommending the most aggressive treatments in order to safeguard against being sued.

payment-centered medical care – Complex regulatory codes that attempt to balance client's rights laws with strict adherence to medical protocol in order to avoid lawsuits and insurance payment limitations designed to contain costs.

health care advocate – Someone who is strong and well-acquainted with the health care system who helps a patient to get the best care possible.

limitation of services – Limitations on insurance coverage and the necessity of spending large amounts of already limited time justifying the need for any treatment not on the insurance company's approved list can lead doctors to not recommend some procedures.

limitation of care – The downsizing of staff has left too few health care workers caring for too many patients. This leaves patients vying for the attention of care providers, and as those providers scramble to keep up it is all too easy to pass the quiet patient by and deliver services to the one who is more vocal, even if the quieter patient needs it more.

health care reform – Reform is needed that balances individual freedom with public good; achieves cost containment through community-based public health prevention programs that remove the causes of disease and provide early diagnosis and treatment to prevent small disorders from growing into large problems; and provides acceptable levels of care and equal access to all, including long term care.

REVIEW QUESTIONS

I.   Completion

Complete the following sentences.

1. A relationship in which one person takes personal responsibility for the good of another person can be described as a _____ relationship.

2. A professional relationship is limited and structured by the existence of very specific _____.

3. The responsibility of the professional to always act for the good of the client is _____.

4. Someone outside of the health care industry who works to get the best care possible for the client is a patient _____.

5. Regulation of third party payees is provided by _____.

II.   Multiple Choice

Select the letter of the choice that best completes the statement.

6. Touching the client only when necessary and only with their permission is respecting
   A. Financial boundaries
   B. Common courtesy
   C. Case law
   D. Physical boundaries

7. Medical care that is based on the good of the client but does not take their rights into account is
   A. Doctor-centered
   B. Emotional boundaries
   C. A helping relationship
   D. Beneficence

8. How to deal with information about the client that is overheard while caring for them is covered by
   A. Confidentiality
   B. Health care reform
   C. Emotional boundaries
   D. Client-centered care

9. One of the major factors that led to the development of client-centered medical care is
   A. The high cost of lawsuits
   B. The civil rights movement
   C. The high cost of medical care
   D. Emotional boundaries

10. Informed consent is a
    A. Financial boundary
    B. Provider responsibility
    C. Patient right
    D. Common courtesy

III.   Matching

Match each term with its correct description.

   A. Nonmaleficence
   B. Client-centered
   C. Emotional boundary
   D. Informed consent
   E. Case law

_____ Maintaining professional objectivity.

_____ Binds a judge to all previous court decisions.

_____ Sees doctors as consultants who provide information and options.

_____ The benefit of treatment must clearly outweigh the risks.

_____ Explaining the diagnosis, treatment proposed, and options in a manner the client can understand and having them sign a statement that this has been done.

IV.   Critical Thinking

11. List some obstacles to health care reform.

12. List some reasons for health care reform.

13. Why do you think client-centered health care led to an increase in medical lawsuits?

14. List areas of medical practice regulated by the state government.

15. Discuss the need for physical, emotional, and financial boundaries.

Section 3
The Client

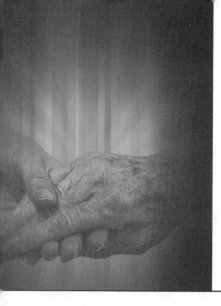

Chapter 8

CHAPTER OBJECTIVES

Upon completion of this chapter you should be able to:

1. Define *loss* and describe the types of loss.
2. List the types of primary losses and discuss their impact.
3. Explain the effects of loss.
4. Differentiate between functional limitation and disability.
5. Define *grief* and list the types of grief.
6. Discuss the impact of grief.
7. Describe grieving behavior.
8. Discuss the purpose of grief and the stages of grief.
9. Define *coping.*
10. Explain the role of experience in coping.
11. Describe factors that aid and hinder learning from experience.
12. Discuss assimilation and accommodation.
13. Define *curing* and *healing* and explain the difference.
14. Describe the gate-control theory of pain as it applies to pain syndrome and disability.
15. List several factors that aid healing.

KEY TERMS

loss	temporary loss	range of experience
internal losses	impairment	depth of experience
external losses	functional limitation	maturity
primary loss	disability	learning from experience
secondary losses	coping	accommodation
sudden loss	grief	assimilation
gradual loss	anticipatory grief	health
anticipated loss	acute grief	cure
uncertain loss	chronic grief	pain syndrome
total loss	delayed grief	gate-control theory
partial loss	suppressed grief	therapeutic relationship
permanent loss	stages of grief	healing

Loss, Grief, and Adjustment

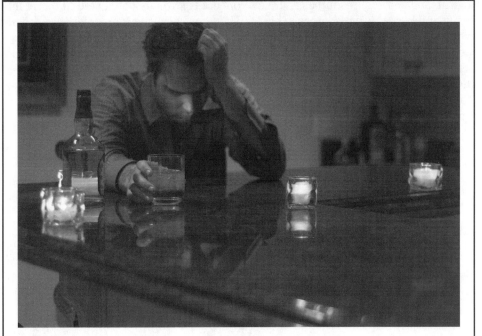

Empathy

The patient has been in your intensive care unit twice in the past with acute pancreatitis associated with excessive alcohol consumption. During his stays in the hospital he has been noncompliant, demanding, and hostile, often becoming sarcastic and insulting to the nursing staff. He has been made aware that the continued excessive use of alcohol will present a serious hazard to his health and his life. When you receive the patient report before beginning your shift you are informed that he is again a patient, has ceased experiencing delirium tremens only within the last hour, and has struck a nurse, leaving bruises. Ten minutes into your shift he presses his call light and with profanity angrily demands pain medication. How do you respond?

INTRODUCTION

This chapter is about the client, what he or she is going through, how it might affect them, and what they need to accomplish.

Look for the definition of loss, the kinds of loss, and the impact of loss. Define grief; look for the types of grief, and the model of the grieving process. Look for the definition of coping and the factors that influence how well we are able to cope. Examine the concept of the quality of life, connect quality of life with people's perception and appraisal of how well they are doing, and relate these to healing.

After studying this chapter you should have a greater appreciation for what client's are experiencing, a better understanding of why they are doing what they are doing, and an increased ability to accept and support their movement through the grieving process.

LOSS

We spend a great deal of time and effort establishing a life that meets our needs. When that life is intact it may include physical, social, financial, emotional, psychological, and spiritual resources. Our self-concept is strongly connected to our ability to put and keep these resources in place. When our basic needs are taken care of and we love and are loved, accept and are accepted, respect and are respected, and when we respect ourselves, we feel capable and worthy. Each of the resources has purposely been put into its place and each plays its part in fulfilling our needs, but none of them stands alone. They are all part of one cloth woven into the fabric of our lives. The loss of one can affect them all, and our self-concept and the quality of our lives can be significantly changed (Figure 8.1).

Loss is the removal of one or more of the resources that a person depends on to meet his or her needs. These may be divided into internal and external and primary and secondary losses.

Internal losses are personal. They may be physical losses such as loss of function of a limb, or mental and emotional losses such as loss of memory, independence,

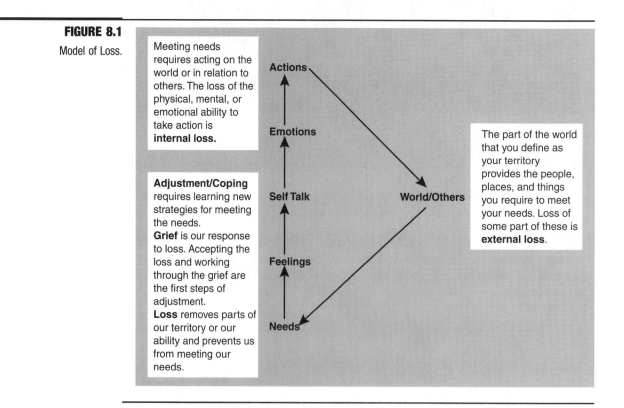

FIGURE 8.1

Model of Loss.

Meeting needs requires acting on the world or in relation to others. The loss of the physical, mental, or emotional ability to take action is **internal loss.**

Adjustment/Coping requires learning new strategies for meeting the needs.
Grief is our response to loss. Accepting the loss and working through the grief are the first steps of adjustment.
Loss removes parts of our territory or our ability and prevents us from meeting our needs.

Actions

Emotions

Self Talk   World/Others

Feelings

Needs

The part of the world that you define as your territory provides the people, places, and things you require to meet your needs. Loss of some part of these is **external loss.**

or self-worth. **External losses** involve the loss of external things such as home, job, or social or family roles.

A **primary loss** is the initial loss. It may be either internal or external, as with a sudden heart attack or the loss of a job. A primary loss can create many **secondary losses**; a heart attack can result in the loss of employment, home, independence, feelings of self-worth, and so on.

Types of Primary Loss

There are eight basic types of primary loss, each presenting a different challenge.

- **Sudden loss.** For example, an unexpected accident, heart attack, or layoff. Sudden loss gives no time for preparation; it can present severe grief and be an acute challenge to one's coping ability.

- **Gradual loss.** For example, the gradual deterioration involved in aging or of a chronic disease. Gradual loss allows much time for preparation and adjustment.

- **Anticipated loss.** We all know what to expect from the aging process, we have witnessed it in the preceding generations. Some diseases have a predictable progression that we can be made aware of and prepare for.

- **Uncertain loss.** Some diseases, such as multiple sclerosis, have a high degree of uncertainty. We can never know when a remission will give way to a renewed onslaught of the disease, or how much or what kind of damage may be done during an acute phase. We must be able to live with the uncertainty and cope with the losses as they occur.

- **Total loss.** For example, the death of a loved one, or learning that you have a terminal disease.

- **Partial loss.** For example, illness or disability that takes away some portion of functioning, or a divorce that reduces us to being with our children only on alternate weekends and holidays.

- **Permanent loss.** Loss with no hope of recovery.

- **Temporary loss.** Loss with good hope of recovery (Drench, 2003).

The Effects of Loss

How serious an impact a loss has depends on all of its elements. The sudden but temporary total loss of employment is not the same as the sudden, total, and permanent loss of the ability to work. Some losses generate a host of secondary losses, others do not. The greater the impact a loss has on our life, the greater the challenge is to our adjustment. All loss creates **impairment** in that it prevents us from meeting our needs. If that impairment limits our personal ability to perform in some way in our life, that inability to perform is a **functional limitation**. If the functional limitation prevents us from carrying out certain roles that are important to us in society it is a **disability** (Nagi, 1965). Franklin Roosevelt had a functional limitation, but he was not disabled. Loss impacts our quality of life and our self-concept. **Coping** with loss requires that we restore the balance and regain our well-being, and the first task is dealing with grief.

GRIEF

All loss creates some degree of grief. **Grief** is a psychological (mind) and physiological (body) response to loss. Powerful loss requires tremendous adjustment and it drives the powerful and confusing feelings associated with grief. As with the function of any feeling, the role of feelings associated with grief is to drive us to make the changes in belief, thought, and behavior necessary to meet our needs. Grief motivates adjustment.

Types of Grief

Grief may be divided into five types:

- **Anticipatory grief.**   Experienced before the actual loss, anticipatory grief involves preparing for future loss; but you cannot adjust to what has not yet happened, and anticipatory grief is associated with greater intensities of anger and loss of emotional control than other types of grief (Gilliland & Fleming, 1998). Those who experience the most anger and hostility, as compared to other family members, tend to be adult children, those not living with the patient, non-primary caregivers, women, and those with more education (Chapman & Pepler, 1998).

- **Acute grief.**   Acute grief begins at the time of the loss. The severity of the grief tends to be directly in proportion to the severity of the loss. The person may experience sadness, anxiety, denial, anger, and depression and may feel overwhelmed, confused, numb, helpless, and hopeless. Acute grief is often expressed by crying and wailing, the inability to eat or sleep, and a loss of interest in things normally found to be pleasurable. The loss can be so great that a person feels as if the world should stop, and often wonders how others can go on as if nothing has happened. Acute grief tends to be associated with diminished cognitive functioning and problem-solving abilities (Caplan, 1990).

- **Chronic grief.**   Perpetual or intermittent mourning. The person does not adjust and may grieve for the rest of their life. This may be due to a lack of ability to adjust in general; because the loss is too great to adjust to; or because the loss never ends, as with chronic and terminal illness or with the parents of disabled children who see a succession of milestones pass, all out of the reach of their child.

- **Delayed grief.**   Grief is held in until a safer moment and then released. Some try to be strong for others, and then break down afterward when they are alone.

- **Suppressed grief.**   Grief is repressed, unfelt perhaps for years, but some future event may unexpectedly trigger its release.

Grieving Behavior

In her landmark book *On Death and Dying*, Elisabeth Kubler-Ross (1969) describes the emotional process involved in dying. Extended beyond the terminally ill, the framework she presents has become a widely accepted model of the grieving process in general. The **stages of grief** she identified are denial, anger, bargaining, depression, and acceptance. It is important to note that this is not a progression but a process. Some may not experience all of the stages, or may move back and forth between stages. Others may not progress but remain in one stage, such as denial or anger.

- Denial.   On first learning of a dramatic or impending loss, it is common for people to try to make it not be true. They want verification or a second opinion, or they believe that by some action on their part they will be able to overcome it. The actions spurred by such efforts are important for the peace of mind of the person doing them, and though they are often futile, they have at times produced remarkably positive effects.

- Anger.   As the reality of the loss begins to sink in it triggers strong emotion. The angry blaming of God, the doctor, the family caregiver, the hospital, or anyone else in a position to be held responsible becomes a channel for this emotion and gives it an outlet. However uncomfortable and unfair this may seem for the one being blamed, allowing this emotion to be released is far better for the grieving individual than bottling it up inside.

- Bargaining.   Following the initial acceptance of the reality of their loss, people often try to make deals with God, promising good behavior or a highly symbolic act in exchange for His intervention.

- Depression.   All of the previous stages represent some degree of non-acceptance of the loss. The goal is for people to work through the process until they are capable of facing their reality without the cushion of denial, anger, or bargains. When they are able to do this, the full impact of the loss often creates deep sadness or depression. This is the time during which they truly grieve the loss. Eventually, the full experience of grief normally gives way to acceptance.

- Acceptance.   Accepting the loss for what it is allows a person to adjust and move past it and focus on what they still have. This can enable a man in a wheelchair to become the President of the United States or a terminally ill patient to enjoy the time they have left, to live until they die.

Modern Grief

Today's world moves quickly. As it sweeps us along like a rapidly flowing stream we have little time to explore the depths, so we respond to the surface. Physical attractiveness and ability are highly valued and grief detracts from these. Employers and others allow only two to three days for grieving. People are supposed to return to their work and social life quickly and be attractive, well-adjusted, and capable. Prolonged grief is seen as a weakness or pathology requiring medical, psychiatric, or psychological intervention, and others quickly lose patience with people's need to process their emotions. Grief is often simply not tolerated, and a person winds up either suppressing it or grieving alone. It can take a year to get back to being reasonably normal after a major loss, and even then sorrow can rise and overwhelm us unexpectedly for years. Make the time to listen. You will be practicing an almost lost art, but as with anything that is rare, it is all the more valuable for it.

COPING

Coping with loss presents a challenge and focusing on that challenge is much easier if it is the only one going on at the moment. If I have financial stability, the support of peers and friends, and if my family is stable and supportive I am free to put my energy into adjusting. If I suffer the disrespect or disregard of my peers or desertion by my friends, or if I have to figure out how not to lose the house, my job, or my wife, my energies are divided and I may not recover as quickly, or as well. But even if I do have to worry about these things I may still recover, for in the end it is my beliefs—about my self, my place in the world, and in life, as well as my spiritual beliefs—that most determine my ability to cope with adversity. It doesn't really matter whether that adversity is illness or disability, the loss of a job, or any of the thousands of other things that can happen to me. It is my ability to cope with adversity in general that either helps or hinders my effort to cope with this one in particular, and that ability is created by what I believe. If my belief leads me to an appraisal of the situation that results in behaviors such as anger, manipulation, inflation of pain, substance abuse, use of defense mechanisms, and non-compliance with health care, my ability to reconstruct a healthy territory is seriously diminished. If my belief leads me to accept the loss without defenses or evasions I will fully grieve the loss, and then I can learn to adapt to the changes.

Experience

My ability to face a major loss and adjust is strongly influenced by both the range and depth of my experiences. **Range of experience** refers to the number and variety of experiences I have had that have challenged my belief system. Have I seen and done a lot, or have I lived in a small and sheltered world? Many small challenges hone my ability to alter my beliefs and adjust, and they prepare me for the big challenges. **Depth of experience** refers to how large my past challenges have been. If I have faced and overcome large challenges in the past a new large challenge does not seem so overwhelming. I know I can do it because I have done it before. It may be true that "if it does not kill me (or overwhelm my ability to cope) it makes me stronger." These two factors, range and depth of experience, contribute to what is sometimes referred to as a person's level of **maturity**, his or her ability to remain in control emotionally and to cope with difficulties. Age gives opportunities to gain experience and mature, but it does not guarantee it. It is always possible to live a long and sheltered life, and it is always possible for a person not to learn from their experiences.

Learning from Experience

Learning from experience means that after we have a particular experience we think and act differently. This is a primary form of adjustment and it requires the same thing that other forms of adjustment do; you must accept the experience for what it is (**accommodation**) without twisting it out of recognition to make it fit into your preconceived ideas (**assimilation**). To achieve this, you must avoid the use of defense mechanisms such as

Denial—Avoiding what you do not want to face

Projection—Blaming someone else

Regression—Acting like a child

Displacement—Taking your feelings out on someone who is not to blame

Emotional insulation—Giving up and not caring

Compensation—Overdoing one thing so you do not have to think about another

Acting out—Impulsively doing hurtful or irresponsible things toward others because you are hurting

(See Chapter 4 for a more detailed examination of defense mechanisms.)

When you accept an experience for what it is, and it defies your beliefs, you are forced to change the beliefs, which changes your appraisals, emotions, and actions; that is, you accommodate the experience. You may not figure it out perfectly the first time, but as each new experience is added to the totality of your experience you make more and more sense of life and develop more and more effective beliefs, appraisals, emotions, and actions. You learn from your experiences and mature.

Adjustment

The World Health Organization (2000) defines **health** as a "state of complete physical, social, and mental well-being, and not merely the absence of disease or infirmity." We spend a great deal of time and effort establishing a life made up of the people, job, house, and community that meet our needs. Once these are in place and we are confident in our ability to get our needs met our world is functional and we are secure. But what if these are in place but we are never confident in our ability to get our needs met? How does fulfilling needs translate into a sense of well-being? Some search for years, alone and lonely, and then find one whom they are able to be happy with for the rest of their lives, while others are never alone but they never seem satisfied. Some live their lives in a wheelchair and find meaning and purpose, while there are professional athletes and celebrities who chase satisfaction as if it were an illusion. At the higher levels of experience, what we need shifts from something "out there" that we must pursue to something inside of us that we must discover. Quality of life is not determined by what we have or by what we are able to do, it is determined by how much we appreciate what we have, as well as the belief and hope that keeps us interested and actively striving toward the future. It is not *what* we achieve that counts, it is *that* we achieve, for with struggle and triumph can come appreciation and self-respect. Our achievement may be that we have put in the hard work necessary and have passed the test, graduated from the school, closed the deal, walked alone for the first time, or for the first time in a year. We may live out our struggle on the large stage of world affairs where we strive to move mountains; or we may live our life on a small and intensely personal stage where we strive to move our legs. The level on which we are striving and how well our needs are actually being met at the moment are not as important to our sense of well-being and quality of life as the perception of how well we are doing (Cunningham, Burton, Hawes-Dawson, Kington, & Hays, 2000). This perception shapes feelings into emotions, determines our level of happiness, and increases or decreases hope, our sense of well-being, how well we comply with treatment, and the effort we put into rebuilding our life.

The ability to adjust to adversity and reconstruct a world that meets our needs is the same ability that allows us to learn from experiences and to construct that world in the first place. If we are using defense mechanisms to cope with our life before it is disrupted we have little ability to adjust to the greater challenge presented by loss.

Healing

The goal of much of medical science is to **cure** the patient, to correct what is wrong; but it is possible to cure the patient without healing them. Pain can be treated leaving little evidence of the original pain-causing condition, but the pain itself can become a self-sustaining "**pain syndrome**" that is resistant to medical treatment (Waddell, 1987). Sensory receptors called nociceptors are activated by pain-causing events. The electrical impulses generated by these receptors are relayed by myelinated fibers to neurons in the spinal cord. The **gate-control theory** of pain (Melzack & Wall, 1965; 1988) suggests that these spinal neurons act as gates that are able to close down or open wide, relaying a range from very weak to very powerful pain messages to the brain. When these pain messages are received in the brain another set of neurons becomes involved that is able to feed messages back to the spinal gate neurons, causing them to stay open, intensifying the pain, or to close, reducing it (Fields & Basbaum, 1999; Weissberg, 1999). These brain neurons are strongly influenced by a person's emotional state. When we are tense and anxious the gates are kept open and pain is intensified. When we are relaxed and calm the gates are closed down and the pain is reduced. Increased pain can cause increased tension and anxiety, further intensifying the pain. This process can escalate until the person becomes inactive and passive. As people get more and more out of shape their muscles become weak, leading to tightness and pain if they try to become more active, generating round after round of anxiety and pain escalation until they are disabled, unable to work or participate in an active life.

A large percentage of patients who visit emergency rooms and clinics for cardiac care have no organic heart disease (Esler & Bock, 2004; Salkovskis, 1992). There is nothing physically wrong with their heart, but they perceive that there is and this perception and the fear it instills can cause them to become oversensitive to chest sensations. The escalating cycles of sensation, anxiety and tension, and inactivity produced can result in disability, without any indication of heart disease.

On the other hand, millions have led full and active lives while suffering from debilitating conditions. Many with terminal illness have found a way to live fully until they die. Pain and illness can often create functional limitations, but it is our appraisal of how well we are doing that most often creates disability. A **therapeutic relationship** enhances the client's quality of life by encouraging acceptance and hope, supporting effort and activity and focusing on what can be accomplished. A person who has adjusted to loss and is actively engaged in life has found **healing**, whether or not they have been cured.

SUMMARY

Everyone experiences loss; it is an inescapable part of life. We may experience the loss of ability due to age, accident or disease, or losses in our world such as the loss of a job or of someone we love and depend on. One loss can lead to others in a cascade that seems to sweep our world from under our feet. Grief is the initial response to loss. It is the first step in our effort to adjust to and overcome the loss. Grieving behavior is wide-ranging and the emotions involved can be intense and unpredictable, but suppressing or otherwise attempting to avoid grief only lengthens and intensifies the effects of the loss. The first requirement for adjustment is that we accept the loss for what it is and work through the grief. This is a learned skill and our ability to do it well is dependent on the same personality factors as adjustment in general. If we are well-adjusted to life in general we are usually able to adjust to serious loss and grief. If we are using defense mechanisms just to cope with day-to-day life we have little ability to adjust to a major loss. Experience also plays a large role in our ability to cope with serious loss. If we have a wide range of experience, and especially if we have lived through deep loss before, we are much better able to adjust to further loss. The truth is that we may never be able to put our world back together the way it was before. The permanent loss of the ability to walk requires not a return to the old world, but the construction of a new one. A person is not disabled because they cannot walk. They are disabled if being unable to walk leads to an inability to function in their life. Many very happy and successful people have had functional limitations, but they were not disabled. Learning to appreciate what we have and build on what we can do is the key to rebuilding a life. Dwelling on what we have lost and on what we cannot do, even dwelling on fear or pain, is a recipe for making it worse and becoming disabled. Some of the most courageous people on earth go unnoticed as they simply and quietly face the day and the pain and effort required to go to bed able to do just a little more, or sometimes just a little less. Even in the face of terminal illness, some find the strength and resolve to fully live each day they are given.

APPLICATION SKILL

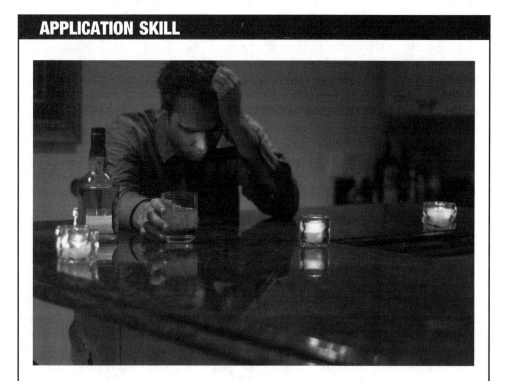

Empathy

The patient has been in your intensive care unit twice in the past with acute pancreatitis associated with excessive alcohol consumption. During his stays in the hospital he has been noncompliant, demanding, and hostile, often becoming sarcastic and insulting to the nursing staff. He has been made aware that the continued excessive use of alcohol will present a serious hazard to his health and his life. When you receive the patient report before beginning your shift you are informed that he is again a patient, has ceased experiencing delirium tremens only within the last hour and has struck a nurse, leaving bruises. Ten minutes into your shift he presses his call light and with profanity angrily demands pain medication. How do you respond?

It is easy to care about some people, with others it is a challenge. Remember that we never know the full story. What can one of us know about the life of another, why they have made the choices they have, or even if they had a choice? We need to search for common ground. Everyone is someone's child, someone's parent, brother, sister, or friend. There is

APPLICATION SKILL (continued)

no one of us that, if caught at our worst, would not disappoint and confuse others. The ability to put yourself in someone else's place, to imagine what you would feel like if you were in his or her situation, can create empathy. Empathy is an objective motivation to help someone else based on an inner identification with their feelings. Sympathy is a subjective sharing of feeling with someone else. To feel sympathy you must not blame them for their own problems or be angry with them. You can feel empathy while hating what they are doing to themselves, yet be motivated to do all you can to help them. Sympathy focuses on wanting someone to feel better, empathy focuses on helping someone to be better. Sympathy might motivate a person to sneak cigarettes to a withdrawing patient with lung disease, empathy never would. Empathy is direct and assertive—you cannot make others' choices for them; but empathy would lead you to do everything you can to help them, including give them direct information about the pain they have caused and the unacceptable nature of their behavior—not out of anger, but out of concern. The difference between independence and permanent disability can be a health care professional who cares enough to simply not take "I can't" for an answer. Truly helping people can be hard and sometimes has nothing to do with making them feel good in the moment. They may not even like you when it is all over, but seeing them actually get better carries a reward beyond whether or not they smile and wave at you. And if they destroy themselves with their own choices, you will know that you did all you could to prevent it.

CONCEPT REVIEW

loss – The removal of one or more of the resources on which we depend to meet our needs.

internal loss – Personal physical losses such as loss of function of a limb, or mental and emotional losses such as loss of memory, independence, or self-worth.

external loss – The loss of external things such as home, job, or social or family roles.

primary loss – The initial loss. It may be either internal or external, as with a sudden heart attack or the loss of a job.

secondary loss – Comes as a result of the primary loss, for example, a heart attack can result in the loss of employment, home, independence, feelings of self-worth, and so on.

sudden loss – Could be an unexpected accident, heart attack, or layoff. Sudden loss gives no time for preparation and can present severe grief that can be an acute challenge to one's coping ability.

gradual loss – For example, the gradual deterioration involved in aging or of a chronic disease. Gradual loss allows much time for preparation and adjustment.

anticipated loss – We all know what to expect from the aging process, we have witnessed it in the preceding generations. Some diseases have a predictable progression that we can be made aware of and prepare for.

uncertain loss – Some diseases, such as multiple sclerosis, have a high degree of uncertainty. It can never be known when a remission will give way to a renewed onslaught of the disease or how much or what kind of damage may be done during an acute phase. The person must be able to live with the uncertainty and cope with the losses as they occur.

total loss – For example the death of a loved one, or learning that you have a terminal disease.

partial loss – Could be an illness or disability that takes away some portion of functioning, or a divorce that reduces us to being with our children on alternate weekends and holidays.

permanent loss – Loss with no hope of recovery.

temporary loss – Loss with good hope of recovery.

impairment – The loss of function that prevents us from meeting our needs, as in "hearing impaired."

functional limitation – Limitation of our personal ability to perform in some way in our life. Due to a hearing impairment, I may be unable to communicate as easily with others.

disability – The inability to carry out our roles in society. My inability to communicate may prevent employment, a normal social life, or a normal personal life.

grief – The psychological (mind) and physiological (body) response to loss.

anticipatory grief – Anticipatory grief is experienced when a loss is imminent and involves preparing for it; but it is very difficult to adjust to what has not yet happened. Anticipatory grief is associated with greater intensities of anger and loss of emotional control especially by adult children, those not living with the patient, non-primary caregivers, women, and those with more education.

acute grief – Acute grief begins at the time of the loss. The severity of the grief tends to be directly in proportion to the severity of the loss. It is often expressed by crying and wailing, the inability to eat or sleep, and a loss of interest in things normally found to be pleasurable. People may experience sadness, anxiety, denial, anger, and depression; they may feel overwhelmed, confused, numb, helpless, and hopeless; in addition, they often have diminished cognitive functioning and problem-solving abilities.

chronic grief – Perpetual or intermittent mourning. The person does not adjust and may grieve for the rest of their life. This may be due to a lack of ability to adjust in general; because the loss is too great to adjust to; or because the loss never ends, as with chronic and terminal illness or with the parents of disabled children who see a succession of milestones pass, all out of the reach of their child.

delayed grief – Grief is held in until a safer moment and then released. Some try to be strong for others, and then break down afterward when they are alone.

suppressed grief – Grief is repressed, unfelt perhaps for years, but some future event may unexpectedly trigger its release.

stages of grief – Denial, anger, bargaining, depression, and acceptance.

denial – On first learning of a dramatic or impending loss it is common for people to try to make it not be true. They want verification or a second opinion, or they believe that by some action on their part they will be able to overcome or reverse it.

anger – As the reality of the loss begins to sink in it triggers strong emotion. The angry blaming of God, the doctor, the family caregiver, the hospital, or anyone else in a position to be held responsible becomes a channel for this emotion and gives it an outlet.

bargaining – Following the initial acceptance of the reality of their loss, people often try to make deals with God, promising good behavior or a highly symbolic act in exchange for His intervention.

depression – Facing reality without the cushion of denial, anger, or bargains exposes the person to the full impact of the loss, which often creates deep sadness or depression. This is the time during which they truly grieve the loss.

acceptance – Accepting the loss for what it is and grieving it allows the person to adjust and move past it and focus on what they still have and on what is possible to achieve. This can enable a man in a wheelchair to become the President of the United States or a terminally ill patient to enjoy the time they have left, to live until they die.

coping – My ability to deal with adversity in general either helps or hinders my effort to cope with a loss, and that ability is created by what I believe. If my belief leads me to an appraisal of the situation that results in behaviors such as anger, manipulation, inflation of pain, substance abuse, use of defense mechanisms, and non-compliance with treatment, my ability to reconstruct a healthy territory is seriously diminished. If my belief leads me to accept the loss without defenses or evasions I will grieve the loss, and then I can learn to adapt to the changes; I am able to cope.

learning from experience – If I learn from an experience it changes how I think and act.

assimilation – Twisting the information presented by an experience to make it fit into existing beliefs. Assimilation can create misinterpretations that often must be supported by defense mechanisms.

accommodation – Accepting information presented by an experience for what it is, even if beliefs must be altered to do so.

range of experience – The number and variety of experiences I have had. The more experiences I have had and the more diverse those experiences have been the greater is the probability that they have challenged my beliefs and forced me to adjust.

depth of experience – Depth refers to how extensively my experiences have challenged my ability to adjust. If I have faced and overcome large challenges in the past a new large challenge does not seem so overwhelming. I know I will live through this because I have lived through terrible things in the past.

maturity – The ability to remain in control emotionally and cope with difficulties. Age gives opportunities to gain experience and mature, but it does not guarantee it. It is always possible to live a long and sheltered life, and it is always possible for a person not to learn from their experiences.

health – A "state of complete physical, social, and mental well-being, and not merely the absence of disease or infirmity" (WHO, 2000).

cure – To correct what is wrong; to remove the cause of disease or disability.

pain syndrome – Chronic and worsening pain in the absence of physical causes. It is self-sustaining pain that gets worse over time until it becomes chronic and debilitating. It may be started initially by acute physical pain or by emotional oversensitivity to normal discomfort, but it transforms into real pain maintained and worsened by anxiety, without any physical explanation.

gate-control theory of pain – A theory that offers an explanation for pain syndrome. Neurons in the spinal cord act as gates to increase or decrease pain messages to the brain. These spinal gate neurons are controlled by brain neurons, which in turn are strongly influenced by the emotional state of the person. Anxiety and tension result in an increase in pain, calmness and relaxation result in a decrease in pain. If anxiety and tension become chronic, pain can escalate beyond medical control without any justifying underlying physical cause.

healing – A person who has worked through the levels of grief to acceptance and has found a way to be actively engaged in life, whether or not they have been cured.

therapeutic relationship – A relationship that helps the person to heal. It enhances the quality of life by encouraging acceptance and hope, supporting effort and activity, and focusing on what can be accomplished.

REVIEW QUESTIONS

I.   Completion

Complete the following sentences.

1. The physiological and psychological reaction to loss is _____.

2. The severity of the losses suffered in the past can be described as _____.

3. The inability to adjust to a loss may result in _____.

4. The purpose of grief is _____.

5. Changing beliefs and behaviors to adjust to new experiences is _____.

II.   Multiple Choice

Select the letter of the choice that best completes the statement.

6. The inability to use your legs is a(n)
   A. Disability
   B. Impairment
   C. Functional limitation
   D. Loss

7. The inability to walk is a(n)
   A. Disability
   B. Impairment
   C. Functional limitation
   D. Loss

8. The inability to work is a(n)
   A. Disability
   B. Impairment
   C. Functional limitation
   D. Loss

9. The loss of my job would always represent what type of loss?
   A. External
   B. Internal
   C. Primary
   D. Secondary

10. The loss of my job because I could not work after a car wreck would represent what type of loss?
   A. External
   B. Internal
   C. Primary
   D. Secondary

III.   Matching

Match each term with its correct description. Terms may be used more than once or not at all.

Internal	Partial	Defense mechanisms	Denial
Anger	External	Total	Pain syndrome
Primary	Permanent	Secondary	Sadness
Sudden	Temporary	Chronic grief	Anticipated

_____ A sports injury that left one permanently unable to walk would represent what type(s) of loss? (Check all that apply).

_____ On learning of a loss, the effort to make it not be true.

_____ The stage of grief in which rage is most likely to be expressed.

_____ Can confuse the grieving process and impede acceptance.

_____ Can intensify and become disabling without any physical cause.

IV.   Critical Thinking

11. Which family members are most likely to express anger in the face of serious anticipated loss? Why, in your opinion, would this be true?

12. Describe several factors that aid and hinder learning from experience.

13. Describe the gate-control theory of pain and discuss the role of negative verses positive thinking in the context of this theory.

14. Why are both assimilation and accommodation necessary?

15. How can a person avoid loss?

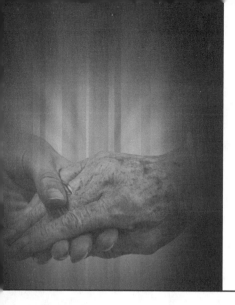

Chapter 9

CHAPTER OBJECTIVES

Upon completion of this chapter you should be able to:

1. Define *adjustment issues*.
2. Define *irrational beliefs*.
3. Define *mental illness*.
4. Discuss the roles of adjustment issues, irrational beliefs, and mental illness as they apply to psychological dysfunction.
5. Identify and describe three examples of disorders identified in childhood.
6. Identify and describe three examples of organic mental disorders.
7. Discuss the nature of substance-related disorders.
8. Identify and describe seven examples of mood disorders.
9. Identify and describe five personality disorders.
10. Identify and describe three types of schizophrenia.

KEY TERMS

psychological dysfunction

irrational beliefs

adjustment issues

mental illness

diagnosis

sign

symptom

attention deficit/
hyperactivity
disorder (ADHD)

autism

mental retardation

organic mental disorders

Alzheimer's disease

delirium

amnesia

anterograde amnesia

retrograde amnesia

dissociative amnesia

mood disorders

major depressive disorder

bipolar spectrum disorder

anxiety disorders

generalized anxiety
disorder

phobia

panic disorder

posttraumatic stress
disorder

obsessive-compulsive
disorder

personality disorders

paranoid personality
disorder

schizotypical personality
disorder

histrionic personality
disorder

dependent personality
disorder

antisocial personality
disorder

schizophrenia

Client Issues

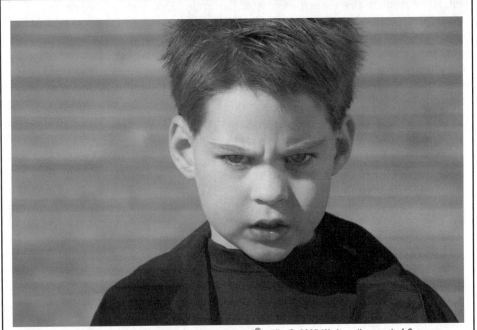

Photo from Plotnik. Introduction to Psychology (with Info TracA®), 7E. © 2005 Wadsworth, a part of Cengage Learning, Inc. Reproduced by permission. www.cengage.com/permissions

Behavioral Modification

The behavior of adults has its roots in childhood, and the dynamics that taught the child have powerful affects still on the adult, especially with the elderly, the ill, the mentally ill, and patients with dementia. Learning to influence the behavior of children is useful in many areas of health care. What is the most helpful way to respond to problem behavior?

INTRODUCTION

This chapter discusses the issues that affect clients as they are seeking medical care. These include the struggle to adjust to loss as well as issues resulting from dysfunctional beliefs and from mental illness. All of these impact the client's approach to the health care provider and their compliance with medical treatment.

Look for the model of psychological dysfunction and identify the roles of lack of adjustment, irrational beliefs, and mental illness in dysfunctional behavior. Also look for the five major categories of mental illness and examples of specific psychiatric disorders within each category.

After studying this chapter you should have a better insight into the nature of psychological dysfunction and specific information regarding a range of psychiatric disorders.

MODEL OF PSYCHOLOGICAL DYSFUNCTION

Most often all we see is someone's behavior. We see what they do, hear what they say. If these things do not seem to us to make sense, or to be acceptable, we look no deeper. But in health care we must look beyond what someone is doing or saying at the moment. There are reasons that people do the things they do; in this chapter these reasons are divided into three large categories: adjustment issues, belief issues, and mental illness. To understand the effects of these we need to expand on the model of psychological processing introduced in Chapter 2 (Figure 9.1).

The part of the brain that identifies a lack of something we require is unconscious (Aurell, 1983). The neurons in that part of the brain register the lack as a need. They communicate this need by producing neurotransmitters and sending them to neurons in the conscious part of the brain. These neurotransmitters create a conscious sensation, a feeling. The feeling is processed with beliefs and perceptions that create an appraisal, which is expressed with self-talk. The appraisal transforms the feeling into emotion. Emotion powers action that is intended to get the original need met. Meeting the need stimulates the unconscious brain to produce neurotransmitters that create positive feelings that stop the action. **Psychological dysfunction** results from issues in this process that consistently lead to behaviors that do not meet needs. These issues are irrational beliefs, adjustment issues, and mental illness.

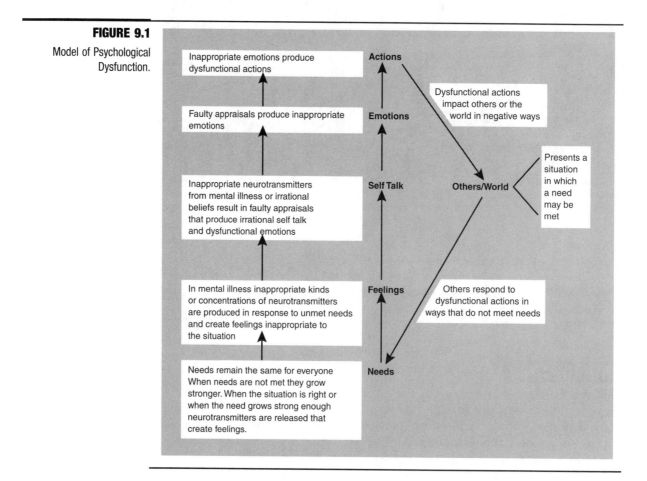

FIGURE 9.1

Model of Psychological Dysfunction.

Irrational beliefs begin as learned beliefs that are used to process feelings. These beliefs create perceptions and appraisals that emerge as self-talk and change feelings into emotions. Beliefs learned in a dysfunctional environment fit well within it, but can be woefully irrational in the larger community. Irrational beliefs produce emotions and actions that are not appropriate to the situation in the larger community and that do not get needs met. Ironically, when the needs are not met, the person quite often blames the community or another person in such a way as to reinforce the irrational belief. For example, prejudice creates behavior that can demean or insult those we are prejudiced against. When they respond to our treatment of them in a negative way we can interpret that negative response as justification for our prejudice. The discomfort and often distress of dealing with the larger world can lead the person with irrational beliefs to create a personal world in which the rational beliefs work. This in effect recreates the dysfunctional world in which the beliefs were formed and passes those beliefs on to a new generation. It can also pass on a legacy of coercion, abuse, manipulation, and violence. Behaviors associated with irrational beliefs may be difficult for the health care provider to accept and respond appropriately to. Prejudice, intolerance, ignorance, or unfamiliar and seemingly counterproductive religious and cultural beliefs can all lead to noncompliance on the part of the client and confound the health care provider. It is important to remember that the patient or the parent of the patient has the ultimate right to accept or reject treatment unless that right has been overridden by the court. A decision to involve the court is made by the physician and should never be made without serious consideration. (For a more complete discussion of irrational beliefs and adjustment see Chapter 4.)

Adjustment issues arise due to changes in the world around us or in our ability to act on the world around us. The loss of the use of my legs impacts my ability to carry out actions designed to meet my needs. A loss in the world removes or changes a person, place, or thing I depended on and prevents me from meeting my needs. In either of these situations I must adjust and learn a new way to do things that will allow me to get my needs met. (For a more complete discussion of loss and adjustment, see Chapter 8.) Behaviors associated with adjustment are the most common issues health care providers face when dealing with their clients. Illness and injury create losses in the client's ability to act on their world. For family members the illness or injury of the client creates a change in their world that renders them also unable to get their needs met. Both the client and the client's family suffer loss and experience grief. Grief is a process of adjustment and until adjustment is accomplished emotions and actions can be powerful and erratic. Health care providers must understand the grieving process and be tolerant of grieving behaviors (see Chapter 8).

Mental illness is at the foundation of the functioning process, where neurotransmitters are created and maintained. It is the result of a disturbance in the production and concentration of neurotransmitters, which can create feelings, thoughts, and perceptions. If I live in constant danger in a world where men roam searching for people to kill, if I see those men searching in the hallway outside of my door and I panic and jump out of the window, even if I break my leg in the fall my behavior is rational and functional in that it may have saved my life. If I have lived my life in a safe world where I am in no danger, yet I still panic and jump out of my window when I see men outside of my door, my behavior is irrational. The wrong neurotransmitters were delivered and they created panic when there was no reason for it. The faulty physical processes that deliver inappropriate neurotransmitters create mental illness, which results in disturbances in thinking, emotions, and actions.

PSYCHIATRIC DISORDERS

Just as with a physical disability, to be a psychiatric disorder, that is, a mental illness, the impairment must be sufficient to create a functional limitation that results in the inability to function in one or more necessary areas of life. The areas most often impacted are employment, social relationships, and personal relationships; but mental illness also often impairs eating, sleeping, the ability to pay attention, and the ability to monitor the environment in order to stay safe. Mental illness has a combination of genetic and environmental causes. The predisposition for mental illness is inherited, and some experience mental illness with no apparent stress in their environment. At the other extreme, anyone who experiences enough stress can become mentally ill, but these are both relatively rare events. By far the most common circumstance involves an inherited predisposition combined with one or more sources of stress in the environment that act as a trigger (Glod, 1998). Whatever the cause, mental illness is at its root a physical disorder in that it involves interference with the production and re-uptake of neurotransmitters in the brain. Remember from the first chapter that neurotransmitters are chemicals made by brain cells (neurons) in order to communicate with each other. Normal functioning requires the production and maintenance of the right neurotransmitters in the right concentrations at the right times.

Many of the dynamics of mental illness make providing effective treatment difficult. One in ten Americans has a mental disorder and one in five will develop a mental illness sometime during their lifetime ("Surgeon General's Call to Action," 1999), but only half of those with psychiatric disorders may seek psychiatric treatment. Many with mental conditions seek and receive care for physical disorders, not for the underlying mental disorder (Silverstone, 1996; Friedman, 1997). Those with mental illness are more likely to have accidents, illnesses, and injuries because they engage in risky behavior and are more likely to abuse alcohol and drugs. For such reasons physical illness and mental illness often occur together, each one making the other worse, and since physical illness is easier to see, it is more often what is treated. The **diagnosis** of any illness is a determination of what is wrong and it relies on the identification of sets of signs and symptoms. A **sign** is a difference that can be objectively measured, such as temperature or blood pressure; it can be identified without the patient's participation. A **symptom** is a difference that is subjectively experienced, such as dizziness or pain; it is felt by the patient but cannot be seen by a doctor. To discuss their symptoms with a doctor a mental patient must overcome the effects the illness is producing on their emotion, mood, and motivation, as well as the stigma often associated with mental illness. Those are major obstacles. Too often all a doctor can identify is the patient's actions, and that may be taken from reports. That is like trying to diagnose appendicitis from hearing that a person was doubled over in pain. Increasing the difficulty is that many psychiatric disorders are episodic; they come and go with no way to know how much time there will be in between. One or more sources of stress in the environment is usually the trigger that brings them back (Glod, 1998), making it seem like the person is using psychiatric episodes as a way to avoid responsibility. If a doctor is relying on reports from parents, teachers, social workers, employers, and so on, these reports can be received from people who may mean well, but who do not understand what is happening. Once a diagnosis is made, providing treatment is often a challenge. Many health care providers who are empathetic with physical illness and pain cannot feel empathy for a client who is as hostile and abusive towards them as the mentally ill often are.

There are over four hundred types of mental disorders listed in the current diagnostic manual, the DSM-IV. This text will summarize some in each of five major categories: (1) disorders identified in childhood, (2) organic mental disorders, (3) substance-related disorders, (4) personality disorders and mood disorders, and (5) schizophrenia and other psychotic disorders.

Disorders Usually Diagnosed During Childhood

As the name implies, these disorders most often make their presence known early in life. This argues for a very strong genetic connection that is expressed as the child begins to develop. In this section we will discuss attention deficit disorder, autism, and mental retardation.

Attention Deficit/Hyperactivity Disorder

There are three forms of **attention deficit/hyperactivity disorder (ADHD)**. The first, attention deficit disorder (ADD), is the inability to pay attention. The second, hyperactivity disorder (HD), is being hyperactive and impulsive. The third, attention deficit hyperactive disorder (ADHD), is a combination of the two. Children with ADD really cannot pay attention. Children with HD really cannot sit still and restrain their behavior. As with all mental disorders, these patterns of behavior involve faulty neurotransmitter production or re-uptake, and the neurotransmitters drive the dysfunction. Due to this, ADHD responds favorably to several related drugs—all of which act as stimulants—that affect neurotransmitters. Ritalin is the most frequently used of these. It increases the effects of two neurotransmitters, dopamine and norepinephrine, increasing the ability of children to pay attention and control their behavior. But there are undesirable effects produced by these stimulant drugs, including decreased appetite, increased blood pressure, insomnia, and headaches. A newer drug, Straterra, seems to offer the benefits with fewer side effects.

Autism

The majority of information we receive from others is not found in their words; it is in their body language, gestures, facial expression, and the tone of their voice. By seeing and hearing these we are able to interpret how someone is feeling and predict what they may do. Something as simple as a smile can tell us that someone is pleased with what we have said or done and can stimulate feelings in us of being safe, accepted, and appreciated. Children with **autism** cannot mentally process this information and so get no information from these things. As a result they are unable to interpret others' feelings or predict their likely behavior. Nothing tells an autistic child that they are appreciated, accepted, or loved. Receiving nothing from others, autistic children collapse into themselves and interact very little. They make little eye contact, develop few or no language skills, and perform repetitive self-stimulating behaviors.

Mental Retardation

Mental retardation is based on a combination of IQ scores and observed adaptive skills in areas such as self-care, safety, home living, social skills, and communication. The average IQ is 100 and the normal IQ range is between 85 and 115. About 2 percent of people score in the gifted range—above 130—and about 2 percent score in the range of mental retardation—below 70. Limitations on the ability to score well on an IQ test and to perform adaptively in life skills can be the result of genetic factors, environmental factors, or brain damage. Limitations produced by an impoverished environment may be overcome if severe neglect has not resulted in an underdeveloped brain (see Chapter 3). Based on IQ scores and adaptive abilities, three levels of mental retardation have been identified.

Levels of Mental Retardation

- Borderline mentally retarded.   About 70 percent of those with retardation fall within this category. With IQs from 50 to 75, they are able to respond to educational opportunities and special training and learn to read and write, become socially competent, learn simple occupational skills, and become partially or completely self-supporting.

- Mildly to moderately mentally retarded.   These individuals have IQs from 35 to 50. With special training they can learn to function with partial independence within a supportive setting.

- Profoundly mentally retarded.   With IQs from 20 to 40 these individuals are limited in their ability to acquire the skills necessary to take care of their personal needs and require supervision throughout their lives.

Organic Mental Disorders

Organic mental disorders are temporary or permanent dysfunctions of brain tissue caused by chemicals or diseases. Discussed in this section are Alzheimer's disease, delirium, and amnesia.

Alzheimer's Disease

Alzheimer's disease is a disease of the aging; in the United States it is the fourth leading cause of death among adults. Ninety percent of the cases begin after the age of 65; the other 10 percent begin between the ages of 50 to 65. The cause of the disease is unknown and there is no cure; the symptoms worsen over the course of five to ten years, and it is always fatal. Symptoms include memory loss, confusion, language deficits, the inability to recognize objects, and the inability to plan and organize tasks (American Psychiatric Association, 1994). The effects of the disease result from the progressive destruction of neurons in the brain. Neurons have an extremely limited ability to reproduce or replace damaged connections, and as neurons are destroyed brain function gradually declines until life functions are lost.

Dementia

Dementia is an abnormal decline in brain function that affects many mental abilities, including memory (see *amnesia*). It can be the result of a variety of diseases such as Alzheimer's disease (see above), AIDS, Huntington's disease, Parkinson's disease, and so on, and it affects 15 to 20 percent of people over the age of 75 (Wise, Gray, & Seltzer, 1999). In the early stage the symptoms include increased forgetfulness and decreased problem-solving abilities. The person often recognizes these changes in themselves and may become frightened by them and embarrassed when others notice and comment. Symptoms of the middle stage include an increased inability to recall recent events and to choose or use the correct word, and becoming easily confused. The late stage is characterized by a pronounced inability to communicate with words or to carry out normal daily activities. As the disorder progresses patients increasingly live in a world constructed by their memory, in which things make sense to them and in which they can get their needs met. As they increasingly carry out physical actions in this world in response to the world in their mind, those actions have less and less contact with the reality around them.

Delirium

Delirium is a syndrome (set of signs and symptoms) produced by recent brain or mental dysfunction. Anything that impacts the brain's ability to function properly may result in this inability to perceive accurately, think clearly, and pay attention. Because it is the result of a recent change in mental status, a diagnosis has to be based on how the person was functioning before the decline. Alzheimer's disease and other forms of dementia may produce the same symptoms but do not represent a recent change. Dementia occurs very often in hospitalized patients, affecting 10 to 20 percent of all adults and 30 to 40 percent of elderly adults.

Amnesia

Amnesia is a disturbance of memory. It can be the result of damage to the brain by injury or disease, drugs (usually sedatives), or of psychological causes such as defense mechanisms or reaction to severe trauma. It may be temporary, permanent, or unpredictable and may begin suddenly or very gradually.

Types of Amnesia

- **Anterograde amnesia.**   Affects the ability to form new memories. The person will retain old memories but will not be able to remember anything that happens after the onset of the disease for more than a few minutes at a time.

- **Retrograde amnesia.**   Affects the person's ability to remember things that happened before the onset of the disease. New memories are formed, but life seems to have begun at the onset of the disease. Retrograde and anterograde amnesia can occur together in one patient. Those with retrograde amnesia often feel embarrassed or stressed by their inability to remember others who identify themselves as family or friends. It is important to take it slow and allow them to get to know you as if they were meeting you for the first time. Just as with anyone else, you should not hug or touch them until they are comfortable with such physical displays of affection.

- Traumatic amnesia.   Occurs usually due to a head injury. Depending on the severity of the injury it may be temporary or permanent and it may be retrograde, anterograde, or both. Trauma such as car accidents often result in the permanent inability of the patient to recall the moments just before the accident, due to a brief interference with the mechanisms that store new memories.

- Korsakoff's syndrome.   Type of memory loss associated with long-term alcoholism or malnutrition. Brain damage results from a lack of vitamin B1 and is progressive as long as the alcoholism or malnutrition continues.

- Alzheimer's disease (see above).   Results in mixed retrograde and anterograde amnesia that is progressive and permanent.

- **Dissociative amnesia.**   Results from psychological causes. It involves the inability to retrieve memories having to do with extremely traumatic or stressful events. Repressing the memory of childhood rape is an example of dissociative amnesia. Since the memories are stored, there is the possibility of recovering them.

- Dissociative fugue.   Extremely rare form of amnesia caused by psychological trauma in which the person suddenly loses the ability to recall some or all of their past, and either loses their identity or forms a new, fictional one and abruptly travels to a new place and starts a new life.

- Blackout.   Short-term inability to form new memories (anterograde amnesia) that may be caused by excessive short-term alcohol consumption or by sedative drugs. This drug induced state may include a blurring of vision and end with a loss of consciousness, but often there is an extended period of activity of which there is no memory afterward.

The drug flunitrazepam (Rohypnol) is a very powerful tranquilizer that produces an effect similar to a large consumption of alcohol, including anterograde amnesia, within 20 to 30 minutes, which lasts for several hours. It is the primary "date rape" drug. Street names include: roachies, rophies, roche, rope, la roche, roofies, ruffies, rib, Mexican valium, and the "forget (me)" pill.

Substance Related Disorders

People have used drugs for at least 6000 years, and continue to do so at an ever-increasing rate. About $140 billion is spent by Americans on drugs every year, with about $91 billion of that amount being spent on illegal drugs (Hanson & Venturelli, 1998). Increasing along with drug usage are drug-related personal, employment, legal, and medical problems that cost our society about $71 billion a year (Schuckt, 2000). Approximately 168 million Americans use illegal drugs each year and someone is arrested for a drug violation about every 20 seconds (Egan, 1999b). Drugs have such a powerful effect on our society because they have such a powerful effect on the individual. Remember that feelings, thoughts, and perceptions are all produced by neurotransmitters and that meeting needs results in neurotransmitters that produce feelings of contentment, pleasure, and so on. In nature this effect is achieved by performing some productive action that helps the person to survive or thrive. The power and problem of illegal drugs comes from their ability to mimic neurotransmitters or block them from being reabsorbed and to produce these feelings of contentment, pleasure, and so on without the person having to perform any productive action. As more and more people have been crowded into smaller and smaller spaces, and as what it takes to survive and thrive in society has become increasingly complex, people have begun to suffer physically, economically, mentally, and emotionally. There is an entire segment of the population who make their way through the crowds every day, but have no one and live alone and lonely; and there are many others who feel the same, even though they share living space with others. Relationships are disposable and friendships are surface and fleeting. Too often we spend all of our energy just to keep our head above water and wind up drifting with no sense of who we are, of what we want, or of where we are going. Even childhood has become a time of pressure to perform and set the stage for the increased pressure of adolescence and the ultimate pressure of finding a place in the large, scary whirlwind of the world. Being born in poverty in a substandard school district is a serious handicap, but relative wealth and a good school do not relieve the pressure. Expectations have soared: the kind of house we must have, the car we must drive, the clothes we must wear, the contacts we must make, the perception we must create, the status we must achieve; and the competition is brutal. Even when we find our place in the world it is too often kept only by increasingly productive performance. In the face of all of that it is no wonder that an ever-increasing number of people choose to feel good now, even if they risk being hurt later. Alcohol, marijuana, opiates, hallucinogens, sedatives, and stimulants are all categories of drugs.

Categories of Drugs

Alcohol depresses the central nervous system, decreases inhibitions, and produces euphoria. The reduced inhibitions make it seem initially like a stimulant in that those affected act on impulses that they normally would not, but the depression of the central nervous system decreases their ability to perform the actions that the reduced inhibitions lead them to. They lose their ability to effectively inhibit their behavior, think clearly, communicate, drive, resolve conflicts, or perform sexually. This leads to a greatly increased risk of rape (including date rape), manslaughter, domestic violence, and accidents in automobiles, at home, and in the workplace. A high level of alcohol consumption is extremely hard on the body and the effects of alcohol abuse are the third leading health problem in the United States, surpassed only by heart disease and cancer. Tolerance to alcohol develops gradually; there is a moderate risk of physical and psychological dependency, and you can die from an overdose, though such occurrences are rare.

Marijuana, hashish, and THC are all products of the hemp plant *cannabis*. They produce relaxation and a mild euphoria along with increased sensory awareness. Tolerance develops gradually but there is no risk of physical dependence. There is a moderate risk of psychological dependence, as well as a physical risk of cancer and lung disease if the plant is smoked. The risk of fatal overdose is low to nonexistent.

Opiates (narcotics) produce pain reduction, constipation, and powerful euphoria. Opiates include opium, heroin, and morphine. These are powerful drugs that suppress the immune system and tolerance to them develops quickly. The risks of physical dependence, psychological dependence, and fatal overdose are all high.

Hallucinogens produce hallucinations that are sensory (visual, hearing, skin sensations, etc.), perceptual, and cognitive (unusual thoughts)—experiences that can be very powerful, but which the person recognizes as not being real. Hallucinogens include LSD, psilocybin from mushrooms, mescaline from the peyote cactus, and a dozen or more artificially produced "designer drugs," such as ecstasy (MDMA), which begin as an amphetamine molecule and then are chemically altered to produce varying effects. Tolerance to hallucinogens develops gradually; there is no risk of physical dependence, and a very low risk of either psychological dependence or of fatal overdose.

Sedatives depress the central nervous system and induce sleep. They produce a relaxed state of euphoria and reduced inhibitions similar to alcohol intoxication. Tolerance develops quickly and there is a high risk of physical dependence, psychological dependence, and fatal overdose.

Stimulants increase the activity of the central nervous system, which results in decreased fatigue and increased alertness, arousal, and can include euphoria. Powerful stimulants include amphetamines, methamphetamines, and cocaine. Nicotine and caffeine are mild stimulants. Tolerance to stimulants develops rapidly. There is a moderate risk of physical dependence and a high risk of psychological dependence, and with powerful stimulants there is a high risk of fatal overdose.

Mood Disorders

Mood disorders involve long-lasting disturbances in emotions that strongly affect feelings, thoughts, and behaviors. Discussed below are major depressive disorder, bipolar disorder, and four types of anxiety disorders.

Major Depressive Disorder (MDD)

Everyone has ups and downs, everyone is sad at times, and sooner or later everyone must deal with grief. These are not the same as depression. Clinical depression lasts at least two weeks, most often much longer, and is marked by its severity. Depression is incapacitating. People lose interest, even in things they normally enjoy very much. They see life as hopeless and themselves as worthless. They cannot concentrate, make decisions, or remember things well. They isolate themselves, cannot eat or sleep well, and can become angry and hostile. Women are diagnosed with major depression twice as often as men. Seventeen percent of all adults, ten percent of the overall population, are affected by **major depressive disorder (MDD)** (American Psychiatric Association, 1994), and suicide resulting from MDD is the eighth leading cause of death in the United States. For every suicide there are eight to ten unsuccessful attempts, accounting for 10 percent of general admissions in hospitals (Weisman, 1998).

Bipolar Spectrum Disorder

Bipolar spectrum disorder affects 1 to 2 percent of the population. Alternating depressive and manic episodes are separated by a period of normal functioning. The depression is major depression as described above. The manic episodes are marked by grandiose thinking and feelings of invulnerability. The person believes they can do anything and loses the ability to accurately assess risks. They display a profound lack of concern for consequences or for their own safety and engage in behaviors that put them at risk physically, financially, and socially. They feel high, are extremely active, talk rapidly and constantly, and display little need to eat, drink, or sleep. Their thoughts can be disorganized, even chaotic, and they may become angry, belligerent, or hypersexual with little regard for the needs or rights of others. At the extreme, they are out of control. More than 50 percent abuse alcohol or drugs and one in four attempts suicide.

Anxiety Disorders

Generalized anxiety disorder produces constant symptoms. Phobias produce symptoms related to a specific situation, event, object, or person. Panic disorder involves repeated and unpredictable panic attacks (described below).

All **anxiety disorders** produce worry with irrational fears and apprehensions that at times escalate to terror. Those with anxiety disorders have an array of aches and pains that have no physical cause, and they intensify discomforts that do have a physical cause. They experience an increased heart rate, shortness of breath, heart palpitations, increased blood pressure, increased muscle tension, nausea, sweating, dizziness, and crawling skin. They have trouble concentrating and remembering things and are very emotionally dependent, constantly seeking reassurance or guidance. They may be unable to sit still and may pace constantly, repeatedly ask for help even when making simple decisions, and can become demanding and controlling. They try to avoid situations that cause them anxiety and worry over things until they turn small problems into insurmountable obstacles.

Types of Anxiety Disorders

- **Generalized anxiety disorder.** It is characterized by excessive or unrealistic worry about almost everything or feeling that something bad is about to happen. These anxious feelings occur on a majority of days for a period of at least six months (American Psychiatric Association, 2000).

- **Phobias.** Fear is the normal response to a genuine danger. With phobias the fear is either irrational or excessive. It is an abnormally fearful response to a danger that is imagined or is irrationally exaggerated. People can develop phobic reactions to animals (e.g., spiders), activities (e.g., flying), or social situations (e.g., eating in public or simply being in a public environment) (American Psychiatric Association, http://www.healthyminds.org/multimedia/phobias.pds).

- **Panic disorder.** It is characterized by recurrent and unexpected panic attacks. The person becomes so worried about having another panic attack that this intense worrying interferes with normal psychological functioning (American Psychiatric Association, 2000).

- Panic attack. Period of intense fear or discomfort in which four or more of the following symptoms are present: pounding heart, sweating, trembling, shortness of breath, feelings of choking, chest pain, nausea, feeling dizzy, and fear of losing control or dying (American Psychiatric Association, 2000).

- **Posttraumatic stress disorder (PTSD).** Anxiety disorder caused by a life-threatening event or series of events that shatter and individual's sense of being able to control a situation and stay safe and secure. The threat is usually to the person themselves but may be to someone they care for deeply. Following the event, those with PTSD have persistent flashbacks, often triggered by people, places, or events that are emotionally charged for them, in which they re-experience the original trauma. These flashbacks are so terrifying that they live in fear and construct their lives around trying to avoid anything that might trigger them, and around trying to avoid risk altogether. Always fearing the worst, they lose the ability to accurately judge what is dangerous and what is not, startle easily at the unexpected, and are constantly on guard against danger. In an effort to shut the emotion off they may become emotionally numb, with a flat affect and even to feel disconnected from reality. They often cannot sleep, become irritable, and have poor impulse control, which ironically may lead them to act in ways that get them hurt, reinforcing their fear.

- **Obsessive-compulsive disorder (OCD).** Affects about 4 percent of people at some point in their lives. The symptoms can stop and start and the severity can change over time. The obsessive part refers to unwanted, uncontrollable thoughts, impulses, or images that interfere over and over again and override people with OCD's normal thoughts and actions. Their brain gets stuck on a track and can't get off. Being compulsive refers to the overpowering drive to perform a behavior over and over again. This behavior is a ritual intended to bring relief from the obsession. If the obsessive worry is over whether or not all of the electrical appliances have been turned off, the compulsion may be to check each one in a specific order a set number of times before leaving the house. If the obsession involves too many sources of worry the compulsive ritual can be so time-consuming as to dominate the person's life and can become a source of anxiety itself. Some of the more common obsessions include:

The excessive need for everything to be in perfect order

Fear of not being able to find or not having things you need

Fear of harming others or yourself

Fear of contamination by dirt or germs

Excessive need of some article believed to bring luck

Sexually explicit or violent images or thoughts

Personality Disorders

Personality is a set of traits that shape behavior. These traits are enduring, that is, they remain the same over time and from one situation to another. **Personality disorders** are sets of enduring traits that shape behaviors that seriously impair functioning or cause severe distress in a person's personal and social life. Personality disorders arise from a combination of genetic, environmental, psychological, and social factors. The development begins with a troubled childhood. Problems developed in that childhood continue into adulthood and result in extremely abnormal behaviors and very poor, maladaptive personal relationships (Vargha-Khadem, 2000). There are six personality disorders (PD), all highly resistant to treatment.

Types of Personality Disorders

- **Paranoid PD.**   From 0.5 to 2.5 percent of people experience this consistent pattern of mistrust and suspicion and the perception that others around them have sinister intentions. They search for hidden meanings in everything and the innocent words and actions of others take on enormous significance as they are twisted into malevolent plots. Battles are constantly seen, and fought, over nothing. They are quick to challenge the loyalty of and shift the blame to others and carry long grudges.

- **Schizotypical PD.**   This disorder involves 3 to 5 percent of people, who deeply mistrust others and are extremely anxious in close relationships. They are most often loners whose distorted thinking and endless rambling off the subject prevents them from communicating. They view themselves as different, sometimes magical; isolated from others. This isolation becomes increasingly painful as they disengage more and more from the world around them.

- **Histrionic PD.**   About 2 percent of the population display this pervasive and excessively emotional pattern of attention-seeking behavior. They are emotionally shallow, self-centered, impulsive, and dramatic, manipulating others with physical symptoms and, especially in women, with suicide threats. Both sexes tend to be sexually provocative and promiscuous, men tend to be bisexual. In close relationships the symptoms worsen, and women in particular may display intense anger.

- **Dependent PD.**   It is characterized by an excessive need to be taken care of that leads about 2 percent of people to be consistently clingy and submissive in most or all of their relationships with others. Those with the disorder have difficulty making everyday decisions without a great amount of support and advice from others, so they find it almost impossible to initiate a project on their own. They insist that others take responsibility for major areas of their life. An exaggerated fear of being left alone and not being able to care for themselves makes it extremely hard for them to disagree with others and they go to excessive lengths to bring and keep caretakers in their life. As soon as one relationship ends they urgently find a way to begin another.

- **Antisocial PD.**   About 3 percent of people, most of them men, disregard or violate the rights or property of others. They can manipulate, lie, cheat, steal, destroy property, harass, beat, kidnap, rape, and kill with no guilt or remorse. They lack what most others call a conscience. Members of this group are often referred to as psychopaths or as sociopaths and they account for many chronic criminals and serial killers (American Psychiatric Association, 2000).

Schizophrenia

Schizophrenia is a serious mental disorder that produces symptoms that interfere with personal or social functioning for at least six months. The symptoms must include at least two of the following: delusions, hallucinations, decreased emotional expression, disorganized speech, or disorganized behavior (American Psychiatric Association, 2000). Schizophrenia is separated into two types, depending on whether the symptoms are positive—distortions of normal functioning, such as delusions and hallucinations—or negative—a loss of normal functioning, such as dulled emotions with little desire to speak or act. Positive symptoms produce no intellectual impairment and respond well to medication, so there is a good chance of recovery. Negative symptoms do produce intellectual impairment and do not respond well to medication, so there is a poor chance of recovery.

Types of Schizophrenia

*   Paranoid schizophrenia.   Affected person may hear voices telling them to do things, or have delusions of being a very important person, or of being hunted or persecuted.

*   Disorganized schizophrenia.   Marked by bizarre ideas and behavior. The person may see their own hands melting, laugh or cry for no reason, babble, or have rapid, powerful mood swings.

*   Catatonic schizophrenia.   Affected person may sit rigid and unresponsive for hours or have periods of wild excitement and activity.

SUMMARY

Clients receiving medical care for physical issues are often also struggling with psychological and emotional issues that can confuse diagnosis, decrease compliance, and complicate care. Most commonly, these are adjustment issues created by the impact of changes in the client or family member's life caused by the loss of health. The health care provider must understand the grief response, be tolerant of the range, intensity, and unpredictable nature of the emotions involved, and support the client, or their family in working through these issues.

Irrational beliefs can be more difficult, as individuals can hold onto these with an array of defense mechanisms. These often involve avoiding responsibility by directing blame and anger toward health care providers. If the health care provider takes these attacks personally the atmosphere created can lead to a decrease in the quality of health care. The provider must remain professional and understand that these issues belong to the client or family member, not to them. The health care provider must not engage in the petty disputes that irrational beliefs and defense mechanisms can create. But not all behavior that seems dysfunctional or even self-destructive to the health care provider stems from irrational beliefs. Unfamiliar religious beliefs may produce non-compliance with or even the outright rejection of modern medicine. Such beliefs are often central to the culture and the psychological and emotional structure of the client. The health care provider must respect the right of clients to their own beliefs and to their own decisions regarding health care. It is the role of the physician to determine if the client is mentally incapacitated and unable to make rational health care decisions on his or her own behalf.

The behaviors created by mental illness are the result of faulty structure and function in the brain and are beyond the control of the client. The health care provider should have a general understanding of the nature of mental illness and of many of the more common mental illnesses. An illness that the provider is unfamiliar with should be briefly researched. Clients are always encouraged toward responsible behavior but providers must take the nature of the illness into account and not allow themselves to react personally to behavior that the client cannot control, even if the client seems to know what they are doing.

APPLICATION SKILL

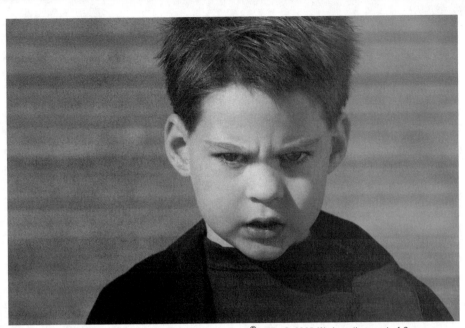

Photo from Plotnik. Introduction to Psychology (with Info TracA®), 7E. © 2005 Wadsworth, a part of Cengage Learning, Inc. Reproduced by permission. www.cengage.com/permissions

Behavioral Modification

Mental illness is at its root impaired physical processing in the brain that prevents a person from perceiving or responding to the world around them in ways that makes sense to others. Due to this impaired processing behavioral modification techniques often will not work as effectively. Still, with appropriate modifications to prevent harm to self or others, they provide a consistent, positive approach that avoids many negative effects.To illustrate the behavioral modification process, let us examine them as they are applied to children.

The behavior of adults has its roots in childhood, and the dynamics that taught the child can have powerful effects still on the adult, especially with the elderly, the ill, the mentally ill, and patients with dementia. Learning to influence the behavior of children is useful in many areas of health care. What is the most helpful way to respond to problem behavior?

Behavioral modification is influencing behavior over time and it takes advantage of the dynamics that form and shape behavior naturally. It is focused on the two prime rules of medicine: "do no harm," and "do good." The first rule, "do no harm," is accomplished by avoiding the mistakes that unintentionally teach irrational beliefs like "I am worthless," or "big people get to hurt little people." Controlling behavior in the moment by force, humiliation, fear, or guilt teaches these lessons and quite often results in a worsening of behavior over time. It almost always renders the person less capable of getting their needs met and living a satisfying life. The second rule, "do good," is accomplished by teaching positive behavior by which the person can get their needs met in productive ways.

Every behavior has a time, a place, or the presence of another person or of other people that make it more likely to occur, and every behavior allows the person to get something they want or avoid something they do not want. Most behavior is social in that it must get the attention of that other person or those other people in order to be successful. Behavioral modification techniques, while not as effective with the mentally ill, still provide the best overall approach. They avoid many of the negative effects of less disciplined approaches, and give the provider working with the mentally ill a compass when they may

APPLICATION SKILL *(continued)*

be at their wits' end. Before you begin to try to change a behavior watch carefully and identify the situation that sets it up and what it is that the person is getting out of it. Once you see these try to avoid the situation that sets the behavior up, and when the behavior does occur pay as little attention as possible to it and do not let the person get what they want to get out of it. Do not let yourself get trapped into responding negatively to the behavior. If it is a behavior you cannot ignore because it is too disruptive, harmful, or destructive, divert the person to another activity or thought or remove them from the situation with as little attention as possible. At the same time watch for the person to do what they should and respond positively to it. Even those with behavior disorders do exactly what they are supposed to do most of the time, but no one notices or responds. The time someone notices and responds is when they do what they are not supposed to do. The cardinal rule of human behavior is, "what you pay attention to grows." Do not berate someone over negative behavior; teach and respect positive behavior instead. If the person gets nothing from negative behavior but gets attention, appreciation, and respect from positive behavior the negative behavior will decrease over time and the positive behavior will grow. Stopping a negative behavior does not help a person to succeed in life and be happy; acting positively does.

CONCEPT REVIEW

model of psychological dysfunction – The part of the brain that identifies a lack of something we require is unconscious. The neurons in that part of the brain register the lack as a need. They communicate this need by producing neurotransmitters and sending them to neurons in the conscious part of the brain. These neurotransmitters create a conscious sensation, a feeling. The feeling is processed with beliefs and perceptions that create an appraisal, which is expressed with self-talk. The appraisal transforms the feeling into emotion. Emotion powers action that is intended to get the original need met. Meeting the need stimulates the unconscious brain to produce neurotransmitters that create positive feelings, which in turn stop the action.

mental illness – The result of a disturbance in the production or concentration of the neurotransmitters that create feelings, thoughts, and perceptions. Inappropriate feelings, thoughts, or perceptions are delivered, and set up behaviors that do not relate to the world around us. One in ten Americans has a mental disorder and one in five will develop a mental illness sometime during their lifetime.

irrational beliefs – Learned beliefs that are used to process feelings. These beliefs create perceptions and appraisals that emerge as self-talk and change feelings into emotions. Beliefs learned in a dysfunctional environment fit well within it, but can be woefully irrational in the larger community. Irrational beliefs produce emotions and actions that are not appropriate to the situation in the larger community and that do not get needs met.

adjustment issues – Arise due to changes in the world around us or in our ability to act on the world around us. As actions are designed to elicit a need-meeting response from the world, either the inability to act, or the removal of the element in the world that would respond to the action, prevents the need from being met. As the unmet needs grow we are put under increasing pressure to learn a new way to act, or to develop a new element in our world, and reestablish the ability to meet our needs.

diagnosis – Illness is a determination of what is wrong and it relies on the identification of sets of signs and symptoms.

signs – Differences that are objective such as temperature or blood pressure that can be identified without the patient's participation.

symptoms – Differences that are subjective such as dizziness or pain; they are felt by the patient but cannot be seen by the doctor.

attention deficit/hyperactivity disorder – There are three forms of ADHD. The first, attention deficit disorder (ADD), is the inability to pay attention. The second, hyperactivity disorder (HD), is being hyperactive and impulsive. The third, attention deficit hyperactive disorder (ADHD), is a combination of the two. These patterns of behavior are due to faulty neurotransmitter production and/or re-uptake.

autism – Children with autism cannot mentally process the information from the body language, gestures, facial expression, or the tone of voice of other people, so they are not able to interpret how someone else is feeling or predict what they may do. Nothing tells an autistic child that they are appreciated, accepted, or loved. Receiving nothing from others, autistic children collapse into themselves and interact very little. They make little eye contact, develop few or no language skills, and perform repetitive self-stimulating behaviors.

mental retardation – Based on a combination of IQ scores and observed adaptive skills in areas such as self-care, safety, home living, social skills, and communication.

borderline mentally retarded – With IQs from 50 to 75, individuals are able to respond to educational opportunities and special training and learn to read and write, become socially competent, learn simple occupational skills, and become partially or completely self-supporting.

mildly to moderately mentally retarded – These individuals have IQs from 35 to 50. With special training they can learn to function with partial independence within a supportive setting.

profoundly mentally retarded – With IQs from 20 to 40, these individuals are limited in their ability to acquire the skills necessary to take care of their personal needs and require supervision throughout their lives.

organic mental disorders – Temporary or permanent dysfunctions of brain tissue caused by chemicals or diseases.

Alzheimer's disease – A disease of the aging that results from the progressive destruction of neurons in the brain. In the United States it is the fourth leading cause of death among adults. Ninety percent of the cases begin after the age of 65; the other 10 percent begin between the ages of 50 to 65. The cause of the disease is unknown and there is no cure, the symptoms worsen over the course of five to ten years, and it is always fatal. Symptoms include memory loss, confusion, language deficits, the inability to recognize objects, and the inability to plan and organize tasks.

delirium – A syndrome (set of signs and symptoms) produced by recent brain or mental dysfunction. Anything that impacts the brain's ability to function properly may result in this inability to perceive accurately, think clearly, and pay attention.

amnesia – A disturbance of memory. It can be the result of damage to the brain by injury or disease, drugs (usually sedatives), or of psychological causes such as defense mechanisms or reaction to severe trauma.

anterograde amnesia – Affects the ability to form new memories. The person will retain old memories but will not be able to remember anything that happens after the onset of the disease for more than a few minutes at a time.

retrograde amnesia – Affects the person's ability to remember things that happened before the onset of the disease. New memories are formed, but life seems to have begun at the onset of the disease.

traumatic amnesia – It is usually due to a head injury. Depending on the severity of the injury it may be temporary or permanent and it may be retrograde, anterograde, or both.

Korsakoff's syndrome – A type of memory loss associated with long-term alcoholism or malnutrition. Brain damage results from a lack of Vitamin B1 and is progressive as long as the alcoholism or malnutrition continues.

dissociative amnesia – Results from psychological causes. It involves the inability to retrieve memories having to do with extremely traumatic or stressful events.

dissociative fugue – An extremely rare form of amnesia caused by psychological trauma in which the person suddenly loses the ability to recall some or all of their past, and either loses their identity or forms a new, fictional one and abruptly travels to a new place and starts a new life.

blackout – The short-term inability to form new memories (anterograde amnesia) that may be caused by excessive short-term alcohol consumption or by sedative drugs.

mood disorders – Involve long-lasting disturbances in emotions that strongly affect feelings, thoughts, and behaviors.

major depressive disorder (MDD) – Clinical depression lasts at least two weeks, most often much longer, and is marked by its incapacitating severity. The person loses interest, even in things they normally enjoy very much. They see life as hopeless and themselves as worthless. They cannot concentrate, make decisions, or remember things well. They isolate themselves, cannot eat or sleep well, and can become angry and hostile.

bipolar disorder – Involves alternating major depressive and manic episodes that are separated by a period of normal functioning.

manic episodes – Marked by grandiose thinking and feelings of invulnerability. Individuals in this phase of bipolar disorder believe they can do anything, and lose the ability to accurately assess risks. They display a profound lack of concern for consequences or for their own safety and engage in behaviors that put them at risk physically, financially, and socially. They feel high, are extremely active, talk rapidly and constantly, and display little need to eat, drink, or sleep. Their thoughts can be disorganized, even chaotic and they may become angry, belligerent, or hypersexual with little regard for the needs or rights of other. At the extreme, they are out of control.

anxiety disorders – Produce worry with irrational fears and apprehensions that at times escalate to terror. Those with anxiety disorders have an array of aches and pains that have no physical cause, and they intensify discomforts that do have a physical cause. They experience an increased heart rate, shortness of breath, heart palpitations, increased blood pressure, increased muscle tension, nausea, sweating, dizziness, and crawling skin. They have trouble concentrating and remembering things and are very emotionally dependent, constantly seeking reassurance or guidance. They may be unable to sit still and may pace constantly, repeatedly ask for help even when making simple decisions, and can become demanding and controlling. They try to avoid situations that cause them anxiety, and worry over things until they turn small problems into insurmountable obstacles.

generalized anxiety disorder – Characterized by excessive or unrealistic worry about almost everything or feeling that something bad is about to happen. These anxious feelings occur on a majority of days for a period of at least six months.

phobia – An abnormally fearful response to a danger that is imagined or is irrationally exaggerated.

panic disorder – Characterized by recurrent and unexpected panic attacks. The person becomes so worried about having another attack that this intense worrying interferes with normal functioning.

panic attack – A period of intense fear or discomfort in which four or more of the following symptoms are present: pounding heart, sweating, trembling, shortness of breath, feelings of choking, chest pain, nausea, feeling dizzy, and fear of losing control or dying.

posttraumatic stress disorder (PTSD) – An anxiety disorder caused by a life-threatening event or series of events that shatter an individual's sense of being able to control a situation and stay safe and secure. The threat is usually to the person themselves but may also be to someone they care for deeply. Following the event the person has persistent flashbacks, often triggered by people, places, or events that are emotionally charged for them, in which they re-experience the original trauma. These flashbacks are so terrifying that individuals with PTSD live in fear and construct their lives around trying to avoid anything that might trigger them, and around trying to avoid risk altogether.

obsessive-compulsive disorder (OCD) – Involves obsessive, unwanted, and uncontrollable thoughts, impulses, or images that intrude over and over again and override normal thoughts and actions; and a compulsive, overpowering drive to perform a set of behaviors over and over again. This compulsive behavior is a ritual intended to bring relief from the obsessive thoughts, but it can become so time-consuming as to dominate the person's life and can become a source of anxiety itself.

personality disorders – Sets of enduring traits that shape behaviors that seriously impair functioning or cause severe distress in a person's personal and social life.

paranoid personality disorder – A consistent pattern of mistrust and suspicion and the perception that others have sinister intentions.

schizotypical personality disorder – A consistent pattern of deep mistrust of others and extreme anxiety in close relationships caused by distorted thinking and an inability to communicate. Those with this disorder view themselves as different, sometimes magical; isolated from others. This isolation becomes increasingly painful as they disengage more and more from the world around them.

histrionic personality disorder – A pervasive and excessively emotional pattern of attention-seeking behavior. Those affected are emotionally shallow, self-centered, impulsive, and dramatic, manipulating others, often with symptoms of illness and, especially in women, with suicide threats. Both sexes tend to be sexually provocative and promiscuous; men tend to be bisexual. In close relationships the symptoms worsen, and women in particular may display intense anger.

dependent personality disorder – Characterized by an excessive need to be taken care of that leads about 2 percent of people to be consistently clingy and submissive in most or all of their relationships with others. Those with the disorder have difficulty making everyday decisions without a great amount of support and advice from others, so they find it almost impossible to initiate a project on their own. They insist that others take responsibility for major areas of their life. An exaggerated fear of being left alone and not being able to care for themselves makes it extremely hard for individuals with this disorder to disagree with others and they go to excessive lengths to bring and keep caretakers in their life. As soon as one relationship ends they urgently find a way to begin another.

antisocial personality disorder – Affects about 3 percent of people, most of them men, who disregard or violate the rights or property of others with no sense of guilt or remorse. They can manipulate, lie, cheat, steal, destroy property, harass, beat, kidnap, rape, and kill without what most others would call a conscience. Members of this group are often referred to as psychopaths or as sociopaths.

schizophrenia – A serious mental disorder that produces symptoms that interfere with personal or social functioning for at least six months. The symptoms may include delusions, hallucinations, decreased emotional expression, disorganized speech, or disorganized behavior. Schizophrenia is separated into two types depending on whether the symptoms are positive—distortions of normal functioning, such as delusions and hallucinations with a good chance of recovery—or negative—a loss of normal functioning, such as dulled emotions with little desire to speak or act, from which there is little chance of recovery.

paranoid schizophrenia – An affected person may hear voices telling them to do things, or have delusions of being a very important person, or of being hunted or persecuted.

disorganized schizophrenia – Marked by bizarre ideas and behavior. The person may see their own hands melting, laugh or cry for no reason, babble, or have rapid, powerful mood swings.

catatonic schizophrenia – An affected person may sit rigid and unresponsive for hours or have periods of wild excitement and activity.

REVIEW QUESTIONS

I.   Completion

Complete the following sentences.

1. Amnesia is a disturbance of _____.

2. Schizophrenia is a serious mental disorder that produces symptoms that interfere with _____ for at least _____ months.

3. Schizophrenia is separated into two types depending on whether the symptoms are positive: _____ functioning, or negative: _____ functioning.

4. Personality disorders are sets of _____ that shape behaviors that seriously impair functioning or cause severe distress in a person's personal and social life.

5. Delirium is a syndrome (set of signs and symptoms) produced by _____.

II.   Multiple Choice

Select the letter of the choice that best completes the statement.

6. In the model of psychological dysfunction, a broken leg would most directly impact
   A. The ability of my world to meet my needs
   B. My ability to act on my world
   C. Appropriate neurotransmitter production
   D. My appraisal of my situation

7. In the model of psychological dysfunction, the death of a loved one would most directly impact
   A. The ability of my world to meet my needs
   B. My ability to act on my world
   C. Appropriate neurotransmitter production
   D. My appraisal of my situation

8. In the model of psychological dysfunction, mental illness would most directly impact
   A. The ability of my world to meet my needs
   B. My ability to act on my world
   C. Appropriate neurotransmitter production
   D. My appraisal of my situation

9. In the model of psychological dysfunction, dysfunctional beliefs would most directly impact
   A. The ability of my world to meet my needs
   B. My ability to act on my world
   C. Appropriate neurotransmitter production
   D. My appraisal of my situation

10. At its root, a mental disorder is a
    A. Psychiatric disorder
    B. Physical disorder
    C. Emotional disorder
    D. Behavioral disorder

III.   Matching

Match each term with its correct description. Terms may be used more than once or not at all.

   A. Neurotransmitters
   B. Feelings
   C. Thoughts
   D. One in one hundred
   E. One in twenty
   F. Are not defensible
   G. One in ten
   H. One in five
   I. The dysfunctional environment that produced them
   J. The world at large
   K. Do not get the person's needs met

_____ A disturbance in the production and/or maintenance of these is the cause of mental illness.

_____ Inappropriate forms of these can be created by faulty neurotransmitter production (include all that apply).

_____ The number of Americans who will develop a mental illness sometime during their lifetime.

_____ Where irrational beliefs are functional.

_____ The ultimate failure of irrational beliefs.

IV.   Critical Thinking

11. Why is it more difficult to properly diagnose mental illness than to diagnose physical illness?

12. Discuss issues that complicate the treatment of persons with mental illness.

13. Normally something that does not work is discarded and replaced with something that does. If irrational beliefs do not succeed in getting needs met, how and why are maintained?

14. Discuss possible effects that failure to adjust may have on the individual.

15. Why is antisocial personality disorder associated with chronic criminals and serial killers?

Glossary

accept To receive another willingly, to respond favorably to him or her.

acceptance Accepting a loss for what it is and grieving it fully allows people to adjust and move past it, and to focus on what they still have and on what is still possible to achieve. This can enable a man in a wheelchair to become the president of the United States or a terminally ill patient to enjoy the time they have left; to live until they die.

accommodation Accepting information presented by an experience for what it is, even if beliefs must be altered to do so.

actions The physical response to an emotion, actions are how we interact with the environment and get our needs met.

active aggression An action intended to harm another either physically or emotionally that is carried out openly either with no effort to avoid taking responsibility or with no fear of the consequences.

active listening Purposely engaging in the process of listening to ensure that you have really heard and understood what the other person is saying.

acute grief Acute grief begins at the time of the loss. The severity of the grief tends to be directly in proportion to the severity of the loss. It is often expressed by crying and wailing, the inability to eat or sleep, and a loss of interest in things normally found to be pleasurable. People may experience sadness, anxiety, denial, anger, and depression; they may feel overwhelmed, confused, numb, helpless, and hopeless; and they often have diminished cognitive functioning and problem-solving abilities.

adjustment Any number of other things can remove elements from the world that a person depends on to meet his or her needs. In order to remain functional, people are required to adjust; to put the pieces back into place and construct a new world that again meets their needs.

adjustment issues Arise due to changes in the world around us or in our ability to act on the world around us. As actions are designed to elicit a need-meeting response by the world either the inability to act, or the removal of the element in the world that would respond to the action, prevent the need from being met. As the unmet needs grow we are put under increasing pressure to learn a new way to act or to develop a new element in our world and reestablish the ability to meet our needs.

aggression Actions that negatively impact another's well-being, used to defend territory.

agreeableness One of the "big 5" personality traits agreeableness describes a person's concern with social harmony and cooperation. Agreeable people tend to be cooperative, sympathetic, trusting, modest, and straightforward.

Disagreeable people tend to be more concerned with self-interest than in getting along with others and can be suspicious, uncooperative, and unfriendly.

altruism The willingness to sacrifice one's own good for the benefit of another. Individuals who score high on the personality trait of agreeableness are genuinely concerned for the welfare of others and are more likely to be altruistic.

Alzheimer's disease A disease of the aging that results from the progressive destruction of neurons in the brain. In the United States it is the fourth leading cause of death among adults. Ninety percent of the cases begin after the age of 65; the other 10 percent begin between the ages of 50 to 65. The cause of the disease is unknown and there is no cure, the symptoms worsen over the course of five to ten years, and it is always fatal. Symptoms include memory loss, confusion, language deficits, the inability to recognize objects, and the inability to plan and organize tasks.

amnesia A disturbance of memory. It can be the result of damage to the brain by injury or disease, drugs (usually sedatives), or of psychological causes such as defense mechanisms or reaction to severe trauma.

anger As the reality of a loss begins to sink in it triggers strong emotion. The angry blaming of God, the doctor, the family care-taker, the hospital, or anyone else in a position to be held responsible become channels for this emotion and give it an outlet.

anger management The development of skills to avoid or redirect anger to prevent it from driving unproductive or self-destructive behavior.

anterograde amnesia Affects the ability to form new memories. The person will retain old memories but will not be able to remember anything that happens after the onset of the disease for more than a few minutes at a time.

anticipated loss We all know what to expect from the aging process, we have witnessed it in the preceding generations, and can anticipate the loss of function and abilities that aging brings. Similarly, some diseases have a predictable progression that we can be made aware of and prepare for.

anticipatory grief Anticipatory grief is experienced when a loss is imminent, and involves preparing for it, but it is very difficult to adjust to what has not yet happened. Anticipatory grief is associated with greater intensities of anger and loss of emotional control than other types of grief, especially by adult children, those not living with the patient, non-primary caregivers, women, and those with more education.

antisocial personality disorder Affects about 3 percent of people, most of them men, who disregard or violate the rights or property of others with no sense of guilt or remorse. They can manipulate, lie, cheat, steal, destroy property, harass, beat, kidnap, rape, and kill without what most others would call a conscience. Members of this group are often referred to as psychopaths or as sociopaths and they account for many chronic criminals and serial killers.

anxiety disorders Produce worry with irrational fears and apprehensions that at times escalate to terror. Those with anxiety disorders have an array of aches and pains that have no physical cause, and they intensify discomforts that do have a physical cause. They experience an increased heart rate, shortness of breath, heart palpitations, increased blood pressure, increased muscle tension, nausea, sweating, dizziness, and crawling skin. They have trouble concentrating and remembering things and are very emotionally dependent, constantly seeking reassurance or guidance. They may be unable to sit still and may pace constantly, repeatedly ask for help even when making simple decisions, and can become demanding and controlling. They try to avoid situations that cause them anxiety, and worry over things until they turn small problems into insurmountable obstacles.

apoptosis Natural, programmed cell death that does not cause inflammation.

appraisal How we size up a situation. It is powered by our beliefs and is the way we processes our feelings and transform them into specific emotions designed to power the actions we have determined most likely to get our needs met. The part of this process we can become immediately aware of is our self-talk, which is an open window into our beliefs.

ask Moving beyond the normal boundaries of conversation and assertively asking for the information and clarification you need to understand the patient.

assertive parenting Making and consistently enforcing rules in the best interests of the child. The child is not included in making the rules because the parent believes that they are in a much better position than the child to know what the child needs.

assertiveness The ability to see what is happening, express your feelings or thoughts about it, and determine your response to it.

assimilation Twisting the information presented by an experience to make it fit into existing beliefs. Assimilation can create misinterpretations, which often must be supported by defense mechanisms.

association neurons The association neuron receives neurotransmitters from the sensory neuron and from multiple other association neurons and makes a decision accordingly. It relays this decision to a motor neuron by sending neurotransmitters across a synapse.

astrocytes Support cells in the brain and spinal cord that tie a group of neurons together by sending out extensions that surround the synapses connecting the neurons with each other. Astrocytes are attracted to the synapses that are used the most.

attention deficit/hyperactivity disorder (ADHD) There are three forms of ADHD. The first, attention deficit disorder (ADD), is the inability to pay attention. The second, hyperactivity disorder (HD), is being hyperactive and impulsive. The third, attention deficit hyperactive disorder (ADHD), is a combination of the two. These patterns of behavior are due to faulty neurotransmitter production and/or re-uptake.

autism Children with autism cannot mentally process the information from the body language, gestures, facial expression, or the tone of voice of other people, so they are not able to interpret how someone else is feeling or predict what they may do. Nothing tells an autistic child that they are appreciated, accepted, or loved. Receiving nothing from others, autistic children collapse into themselves and interact very little. They make little eye contact, develop few or no language skills, and perform repetitive self-stimulating behaviors.

autonomic Motor neurons that take electrical impulses to glands and to involuntary muscle in the heart, organs, and blood vessels. The autonomic nervous system is subdivided into the sympathetic and the parasympathetic divisions.

awareness Paying attention to and becoming aware of negative self-talk, irrational beliefs, and defense mechanisms enables a person to identify when they are using them, and to choose not to.

axons Fibers that carry electrical impulses away from the cell body.

bargaining Following the initial acceptance of the reality of their loss, people often try to make deals with God, promising good behavior or a highly symbolic act in exchange for His intervention.

behavior The set of emotions and actions that flow from feelings. It is the effort expended in the attempt to meet a need.

behavior activation center The association area in the cerebrum that assumes that behavior will be successful and causes actions to be performed.

behavior inhibition center The association area in the cerebrum that assumes that behavior will not be successful, initiates doubt, and stops behavior from being performed.

behavioral modification Influencing behavior over time.

beneficence Do good; all that is done should be done for the good of the patient.

bias Perceiving a person as lesser based on a stigma.

bipolar spectrum disorder Involves alternating major depressive and manic episodes that are separated by a period of normal functioning.

blackout Short-term inability to form new memories (anterograde amnesia) that may be caused by excessive short-term alcohol consumption or by sedative drugs.

borderline mentally retarded Individuals with IQs from 50 to 75 are able to respond to educational opportunities and special training and learn to read and write, become socially competent, learn simple occupational skills, and become partially or completely self-supporting.

brain Encased in the skull, the brain is the central processing unit for electrical impulses coming in from sensory neurons and going out by motor neurons. It may be divided by structure and what that structure enables the body to do, and by function and how that function allows the person to interact with the environment.

brain stem The central core and base of the brain, the brain stem carries out processes vital to the physical well-being and survival of the body. It connects the rest of the brain to the spinal cord.

case law Established by legal interpretations of medical regulations as medical questions are brought before the court. New interpretations can be made with any case and these interpretations establish new law as all judges afterward are bound to them unless they are overturned by the state or federal Supreme Court.

catatonic schizophrenia An affected person may sit rigid and unresponsive for hours or have periods of wild excitement and activity.

cell body The bulk of the cell; contains the DNA and cell machinery.

central nervous system The brain and spinal cord.

cerebellum The cerebellum coordinates the activities of voluntary muscle.

cerebrum The cerebrum is the largest part of the brain and is responsible for awareness of physical sensations, voluntary responses, and sight. It is the seat of higher mental functions such as creativity, art, analytical thinking, and mathematics; and it contains the behavior activation and behavior inhibition centers.

change Paying attention to and becoming aware of positive self-talk and rational beliefs allows people to practice using them in their imagination and to identify and try to perform behaviors based on them. The more people imagine, and the more they try, the faster their brain figures out what they are trying to do and what connections are necessary to make it work. When the new connections have grown new abilities are created. The connections respond to continued use by becoming ever more efficient and effective, thus creating change.

character deficits A perceived psychological or behavioral difference that lowers a person's status. Character deficits may include such things as honesty, ambition, and aggressiveness.

character stigma (this will replace character deficits) A perceived psychological or behavioral difference that lowers a person's status. Character stigmas may include such things as dishonesty, disloyalty, and aggressiveness.

chemical consciousness The contemporary scientific view is that consciousness is the result of patterns and concentrations of neurotransmitters (chemicals) in the brain.

chronic grief Perpetual or intermittent mourning. The person does not adjust to a loss and may grieve for the rest of his or her life. This may be due to a lack of ability to adjust in general; because the loss is too great to adjust to; or because the loss never ends, as with the parents of disabled children who see a succession of milestones pass, all out of the reach of their child.

client-centered medical care With the client as the center, the doctor is seen as a consultant who provides information and advice, but the patient makes the decisions. The patient becomes a client who can shop around, consulting different doctors until they get an answer they like.

coercion The use force or the realistic threat of force to get children to do what the parent wants. It is always accompanied by either physical or emotional abuse, because threats alone lose their power in time if the child is not either hurt occasionally or hurt severely enough initially to leave a permanent impression.

cognitive stages The brain moves through four stages of development, focused on specific developmental tasks, in order to give the child time to experience the world and master simple tasks first before moving on to more complex ones at each level.

collectivist culture Values conformity to group values and rules and there is considerable pressure on individuals to conform to shared beliefs and behaviors. There is a large safety net and a wide range of needs are provided for should a person not be capable of providing for themselves.

communication The art of accurately transferring meaning from one person to another.

concrete functions The cognitive stage from 7 to 11 years. Logic and reason develop and are used in a black or white manner, dealing with what is present in the moment in order to gain what is wanted or avoid what is not wanted. Approval, affection, and acceptance are sought from those holding power in the family and in the group. Sexuality develops.

conditional parenting Means, "I like you and I love you if you do what I want, but I do not like you and I do not love you if you do not. No matter how hard a child tries, he or she can never please the parent all the time, and the inevitable rejection soon teaches the child that he or she is worth nothing inherently; it is only what his or she is seen to do that matters.

confidentiality Clients have the right to confidentiality. Anything you learn about the client is given to you in trust, and information about a client, either medical or personal, even the fact that the client is at your facility, can never be shared without the client's written permission.

conscientiousness One of the "big 5" personality traits conscientiousness reflects the way we control our impulses. Conscientious people tend to be disciplined and well organized, diligent, punctual, and dependable. A low score on conscientiousness indicates impulsiveness, which places more importance on immediate rather than delayed gratification and can be destructive to a person's personal, social, and professional relationships.

consciousness Awareness, including self-awareness.

coping Our ability to deal with adversity in general either helps or hinders our efforts to cope with a loss, and that ability is created by what we believe. If our beliefs lead us to an appraisal of the situation that results in behaviors such as anger, manipulation, inflation of pain, substance abuse, use of defense mechanisms, and non-compliance to treatment, our ability to reconstruct a healthy territory is seriously diminished. If our beliefs lead us to accept a loss without defenses or evasions, we will grieve the loss fully, and then we can learn to adapt to the changes; we are able to cope.

courtesy Clients have the right to be treated with courtesy and respect. Harsh, demeaning, or harassing actions or words by health care providers are never appropriate.

culture The values, traditions, belief system, and practices of a community of people.

cure To correct what is wrong; to remove the cause of disease or disability.

decisions All of the neurons with which one neuron is connected have input into the decisions the neuron makes. A neuron says to another neuron, "yes, do that," by sending one or more neurotransmitters to it across a synapse. A neuron says to another neuron, "no, don't do that," by sending one or more neuroinhibitors to it across a synapse. If a neuron receives more neurotransmitters than neuroinhibitors from the other neurons with which it is connected it generates an electrical impulse.

defense mechanisms Dysfunctional behaviors that do not meet our needs can be locked into repetitive patterns by irrational beliefs, and the belief system is challenged by the question: "Why can I not get my needs met?" Efforts to avoid this question or explanations manufactured to evade personal responsibility for it are defense mechanisms.

defensive medicine By the early 1970's many doctors were responding to the increased number of lawsuits that resulted from client-centered medical care by suggesting every conceivable diagnostic procedure and recommending the most aggressive treatments in order to safeguard against being sued.

delayed grief Grief is held in until a safer moment and then released. Some try to be strong for others, and then break down afterward when they are alone.

delirium A syndrome (set of signs and symptoms) produced by recent brain or mental dysfunction. Anything that impacts the brain's ability to function properly may result in this inability perceive accurately, think clearly, and pay attention.

dendrites Fibers that carry electrical impulses to the cell body.

denial On first learning of a dramatic or impending loss it is common for people to try to make it not be true. They want verification or a second opinion, or they believe that by some action on their part they will be able to overcome or reverse it.

dependent personality disorder Characterized by an excessive need to be taken care of that leads about 2 percent of people to be consistently clingy and submissive in most or all of their relationships with others. Those with the disorder have difficulty making everyday decisions without a great amount of support and advice from others, so they find it almost impossible to initiate a project on their own. They insist that others take responsibility for major areas of their life. An exaggerated fear of being left alone and not being able to care for themselves makes it extremely hard for them to disagree with others, and they go to excessive lengths to bring and keep caretakers in their life. As soon as one relationship ends they urgently find a way to begin another.

depression Facing reality without the cushion of denial, anger, or bargains exposes people to the full impact of a loss, which often creates deep sadness or depression. This is the time during which they truly grieve the loss (see also Major Depressive Disorder).

depth of experience Depth refers to how extensively our experiences have challenged our ability to adjust. If we have faced and overcome large challenges in the past, a new large challenge does not seem so overwhelming. We know we will live through this because we have lived through terrible things in the past.

diagnosis Illness is a determination of what is wrong. and it relies on the identification of sets of signs and symptoms.

diencephalon The diencephalon contains the thalamus and the hypothalamus and is the major switchboard of the brain, sending all impulses to their proper locations. It is also responsible for the body's automatic physical processes and for the mind-body connection.

disability The inability to carry out roles that are important to us in society. For example an inability to communicate may prevent employment or a satisfying social or personal life.

discrimination A difference in how a person is treated based on a belief or prejudice rather than individual characteristics.

disorganized schizophrenia Marked by bizarre ideas and behavior. The person may see their own hands melting, laugh or cry for no reason, babble, or have rapid, powerful mood swings.

dissociative amnesia Results from psychological causes. It involves the inability to retrieve memories having to do with extremely traumatic or stressful events.

dissociative fugue Extremely rare form of amnesia caused by psychological trauma in which people suddenly lose the ability to recall some or all of their past and either lose their identity or form a new, fictional one and abruptly travels to a new place and start a new life.

divisions of nervous system The nervous system has three primary divisions composed of three types of neurons: sensory, association, and motor.

DNA The genetic material inside of cells that contains the plans for making and running the body.

doctor-centered medical care Until the 1960s, doctors were seen as the experts and most people followed their directions without question. This was based on the good of the client, but not their rights. Information was often withheld, treatments could be forced, and involuntary commitment was relatively simple, all based solely on the doctor's evaluation.

domain A group of neurons tied together by one astrocyte. An astrocyte has the ability to override the normal neurotransmitter/neuroinhibitor balance and cause all of the neurons in its domain to generate electrical impulses at the same time. Synapses and neurons that are used too little can degenerate, wither, and die. The effect of this process is to speed and strengthen functions that are used and eliminate functions that are not used.

dysfunctional Beliefs and behaviors produce a response in others that does not meet our needs.

emotional boundaries Involve objectivity. Compassion and care cannot be allowed to cloud professional judgment.

emotional development Erik Erikson described set of eight emotional **dilemmas** that must be resolved as we grow. The way we resolve these determines our feelings, which create the foundation for our emotions and actions.

emotions Feelings that have been processed and modified by beliefs. Emotions are designed to drive actions.

empathy A motivation to help others based on an inner identification with their feelings. Empathy can be created by the ability to mentally put yourself in their place, to feel what it would be like if you were in their situation.

encouragement To inspire someone with courage or hope; to support them.

environment The immediate world that surrounds a person. People, location, buildings, schools, automobiles, economy, animals, culture, and position are all elements of the environment and all have an affect on the development of the child. They determine how the genetic plan will be expressed and the final form of personality traits.

Erikson's emotional dilemmas Erik Erikson proposed a set of eight emotional dilemmas that each person must resolve as part of the development process. These dilemmas exist as a set of extremes, and the individual will become established at some point on a continuum between the two. The point at which a person becomes established is determined by genetic predisposition and interactions with the environment. Erikson's dilemmas are trust versus mistrust; autonomy versus doubt and shame; initiative versus guilt; industry versus inferiority; identity versus role confusion; intimacy versus isolation; generativity versus self-absorption; and integrity versus despair.

ethnocentrism The belief that one's culture's values, beliefs, and practices are the right ones, which makes others who do not share those values, beliefs, and practices wrong.

external loss The loss of external things such as home, job, or social or family roles.

extraversion One of the "big 5" personality traits extraversion describes a person's engagement with the world. People who score high in extraversion are emotionally positive and energetic; they tend to be upbeat, friendly, outgoing, sociable, and assertive and they like attention. Those who score low lack this energy and activity level. They tend to be quiet, low-key, deliberate, and independent, preferring to be alone.

federal regulations Govern third-party payees such as insurance companies, health maintenance organizations, Medicaid, and Medicare.

feelings A conscious awareness of a need.

fight-or-flight reactions Emergency or stress responses during which the heart beats faster and harder; the blood supply to the heart and to voluntary (skeletal) muscle increases; the blood supply to digestion decreases; breathing becomes faster and deeper; sweating increases; and glucose is made readily available for energy production.

financial boundaries Involve payment. Professionals are paid to apply their skill. Without payment a professional relationship does not exist.

five trait personality theory Robert McCrae and Paul Costa have identified five traits that can be measured to describe personality. These traits represent an extreme of personality and each has an opposite. The trait a person develops will establish itself somewhere along the continuum between the two extremes. The point on the continuum at which a person becomes established is determined by genetic predisposition and interactions with the environment. These five personality traits are extraversion, agreeableness, conscientiousness, neuroticism, and openness to experience.

formal operations Cognitive stage at 12+ years. Higher mental functions requiring abstract thought emerge. The ability to understand and use principles, think through alternatives, and base behavior on beliefs of what should be develops. Needs for recognition and respect from others grow into the need for self-respect, requiring motivation and direction from within.

fraternal twins Twins who develop from separate eggs who are related genetically simply as siblings.

functional Beliefs and behaviors influence others in our environment to respond in such a way as to meet our needs.

functional divisions of the brain Functionally, the brain may be divided into the brain stem, the reptilian complex, the limbic system, and the neocortex.

functional limitation Limitation of our personal ability to perform in some way in our life. For example, due to a hearing impairment a person may be unable to communicate with others.

gate-control theory of pain A theory that offers an explanation for pain syndrome. Neurons in the spinal cord act as gates to increase or decrease pain messages to the brain. These spinal gate neurons are controlled by brain neurons that in turn are strongly influenced by the emotional state of the person. Anxiety and tension result in an increase in pain; calmness and relaxation result in a decrease in pain. If anxiety and tension become chronic, pain can escalate beyond medical control without any justifying underlying physical cause.

generalized anxiety disorder Characterized by excessive or unrealistic worry about almost everything or feeling that something bad is about to happen. These anxious feelings occur on a majority of days for a period of at least six months.

genetic plans In the DNA present the model for the development of the body and the brain and for each personality trait.

gradual loss The gradual deterioration involved in aging or of a chronic disease. Gradual loss allows much time for preparation and adjustment.

grief The psychological (mind) and physiological (body) response to loss.

healing Healing occurs when a person has worked through the levels of grief to acceptance and has found a way to be actively engaged in life, whether or not he or she has been cured.

health A "state of complete physical, social, and mental well-being, and not merely the absence of disease or infirmity" (WHO, 2000).

health care advocate Someone who is strong and well-acquainted with the health care system who helps a patient to get the best care possible.

health care reform Needed that balances individual freedom with public good; achieves cost containment through community-based public health prevention programs that remove the causes of disease and provide early diagnosis and treatment to prevent small disorders from growing into large problems; and provides acceptable levels of care and equal access to all, including long-term care.

helping relationship One in which one person takes the responsibility for doing what is in the best interests of another.

history of caring Humankind has a long history of caring for those in need. Early modern human and Neanderthal burials excavated from over 100,000 years ago reveal healed areas on bones that would have been devastating breaks and that would have required the care and support of others for the individual to have survived long enough to heal.

history of health care There have been three distinct philosophies that have governed the provision of health care through the years. These might be characterized as the doctor-centered, client-centered, and payment-centered phases.

histrionic personality disorder A pervasive and excessively emotional pattern of attention-seeking behavior. Those affected are emotionally shallow, self-centered, impulsive, and dramatic, manipulating others, often with symptoms of illness and, especially in women, with suicide threats. Both sexes tend to be sexually provocative and promiscuous, men tend to be bisexual. In close relationships the symptoms worsen, and women in particular may display intense anger.

identical twins Twins who develop from one fertilized egg and have identical DNA.

impairment A loss of function that prevents us from meeting certain needs, as in "hearing impaired."

individualistic culture Values independence and personal responsibility. Individuals are given a great degree of autonomy and freedom but are seen as being responsible for meeting their own needs. There is little safety net with only very basic needs provided for should a person not be capable of providing for themselves.

indulgence Giving children no limits. Their parents either allow them to do as they please or make only feeble attempts at control, giving in whenever the child pleads or has tantrums. In addition, the parent most often protects the child when they get into trouble in the community, refusing to allow them to experience the consequences of their own behavior.

informed consent The client's right to be informed of their diagnosis in a language they understand, what treatment is being proposed, the possible risks and benefits of the proposed treatment and of non-treatment, and of reasonable alternatives to the proposed treatment. Clients must sign a statement indicating that these things have been explained to them, that they understand them, and that they accept the proposed treatment.

institutionalized discrimination When biased beliefs are shared across a culture and lead to a reduced access to goods, services, and opportunities that is enforced openly by overt law or hidden in covert policy or practice.

interactions How thoroughly the genetic plan is implemented depends on interactions with the environment. The final personality traits are influenced both by heredity and by the environment. Personality traits strongly tend to be enduring because they are locked into the physical structure of the brain.

internal loss Personal physical losses such as loss of a limb or function, or mental and emotional losses such as loss of memory, independence, or self-worth.

internalized discrimination The tendency of a person raised as a victim of discrimination to see themselves as undeserving of the same goods, services, or opportunities as others.

irrational beliefs Dysfunctional, as they lead to negative self-talk that promotes defense mechanisms, which block adjustment.

Kohlberg's moral levels Maslow's hierarchy establishes multiple levels of needs that must be met in order. Over time, the lowest level need that is consistently unmet grows ever more powerful until it motivates thoughts, emotions, and actions at that level. This motivation is the key to moral levels. Moral levels are defined not by what we do, but by why we do it. As the lowest order need that is chronically unmet grows powerful, it motivates behavior that can often be described by the characteristics of the moral at that level.

Korsakoff's syndrome A type of memory loss associated with long-term alcoholism or malnutrition. Brain damage results from a lack of vitamin B1 and is progressive as long as the alcoholism or malnutrition continues.

learning from experience If we learn from an experience it changes how we think and act.

limbic system Developed after the reptilian complex, the limbic system motivates and guides group behavior by facilitating emotion, memory, and motivation.

limitation of care The downsizing of staff has left too few health care workers caring for too many patients. This leaves patients vying for the attention of care providers, and as those providers scramble to keep up it is all too easy to pass the quiet patient by and deliver services to the one who is more vocal, even if the quieter patient needs it more.

limitation of services Limitations on insurance coverage and the necessity of spending large amounts of already limited time justifying the need for any treatment not on the insurance company's approved list can lead doctors to not recommend some procedures.

listen Active listening is purposely engaging in the process of listening to ensure that you have really heard and understood what the other person is saying.

look The primary method of gathering information about others, it utilizes an extensive development in the brain devoted to gathering and interpreting non-verbal information.

loss The removal of one or more of the resources that we depend on to meet our needs.

major depressive disorder (MDD) Clinical depression lasts at least two weeks, most often much longer, and is marked by its incapacitating severity. People lose interest, even in things they normally enjoy very much. They see life as hopeless and themselves as worthless. They cannot concentrate, make decisions, or remember things well. They isolate themselves, cannot eat or sleep well, and can become angry and hostile.

manic episodes Marked by grandiose thinking and feelings of invulnerability. People in this phase of bipolar disorder believe they can do anything, and lose the ability to accurately assess risks. They display a profound lack of concern for consequences or for their own safety and engage in behaviors that put them at risk physically, financially, and socially. They feel high, are extremely active, talk rapidly and constantly, and display little need to eat, drink, or sleep. Their thoughts can be disorganized, even chaotic, and they may become angry, belligerent, or hypersexual with little regard for the needs or rights of others. At the extreme, they are out of control.

Maslow's hierarchy of needs Abraham Maslow proposed that needs exist in an order from lowest to highest, and that lower needs must be fulfilled before higher needs can emerge. These needs are physical, safety and security, love and belonging, self-esteem, and self-actualization. The lowest need that is not adequately fulfilled will grow to dominate as neurotransmitters are produced creating feelings that drive the person toward fulfilling the need.

maturity The ability to remain in control emotionally and to cope with difficulties. Age gives opportunities to gain experience and mature, but it does not guarantee it. It is always possible to live a long and sheltered life, and it is always possible for people not to learn from their experiences.

medical ethics Rules that regulate the practice of medicine with regard to patient rights and provider responsibilities.

mental illness The result of a disturbance in the production or concentration of the neurotransmitters that create feelings, thoughts, and perceptions. The wrong feelings, thoughts, or perceptions are delivered and set up behaviors that do not relate to the world around us. One in ten Americans has a mental disorder and one in five will develop a mental illness sometime during their lifetime.

mental retardation Based on a combination of IQ scores and observed adaptive skills in areas such as self-care, safety, home living, social skills, and communication.

metaphysics Reality and rules beyond the limits of our universe and our understanding. Science and religion both recognize the existence of this reality.

mildly to moderately mentally retarded These individuals have IQs from 35 to 50. With special training they can learn to function with partial independence within a supportive setting.

model of psychological dysfunction The part of the brain that identifies a lack of something we require is unconscious. The neurons in that part of the brain register the lack as a need. They communicate this need by producing neurotransmitters and sending them to neurons in the conscious part of the brain. These neurotransmitters create a conscious sensation, a feeling. The feeling is processed with beliefs and perceptions that create an appraisal, which is expressed by self-talk. The appraisal transforms the feeling into emotion. Emotion powers action that is intended to get the original need met. Meeting the need stimulates the unconscious brain to produce neurotransmitters that create positive feelings that stop the action.

mood disorders Involve long-lasting disturbances in emotions that strongly affect feelings, thoughts, and behaviors.

moral levels Moral levels are defined not by what we do, but by why we do it. As the lowest order need that is chronically unmet grows powerful, it motivates behavior that can most often be defined and predicted by the morals at that level.

motor nervous system The motor neurons are divided into two groups, the somatic and the autonomic divisions.

motor neurons Motor neurons receive electrical impulses from association neurons and take those impulses out into the body to an effector—a muscle or a gland.

multiculturalism Today's world is a multicultural mix with new arrivals every day, bringing together people with widely different customs, values, and beliefs.

myelin sheath A covering wrapped around some nerve fibers that greatly increases the speed of electrical impulses.

necrosis Unnatural cell death due to disease or injury that does cause inflammation.

needs All that we require to survive and thrive

needs correlated with moral levels

Physical needs	Power
Safety & security	Deals
Love	Good boy/good girl
Belonging	Rules (authority)
Esteem	Social contracts
Self-actualization	Individual conscience

neglect A parenting style in which the parent has the consistent tendency to ignore the child. Neglectful parenting does not take care of the child's physical needs, but more than that it does not give the child the ability to interact with the world in order to generate growth and development of the brain; neurons that are not used die and go away, forever limiting the child's future potential.

neocortex The latest and most complex development in the brain, the neocortex is responsible for the higher mental functions that we identify with being human and humane.

nerves Long bundles of fibers that carry electrical impulses in the peripheral nervous system.

neurodevelopment The growth and organization of the nervous system. Without interaction with the environment, much of this development does not take place; or if it has taken place, the connections and neurons quickly degenerate.

neuroinhibitors Chemicals that stop electrical impulses from being passed from one neuron to another across a synapse.

neurons The working cells of the nervous system that conduct electrical impulses and make decisions.

neuroticism One of the "big 5" personality traits neuroticism describes a person's tendency to have negative feelings. People who are emotionally negative tend to be anxious, hostile, insecure, vulnerable, and self-conscious. People who score low in neuroticism tend to be emotionally stable, secure, and calm.

neurotransmitters Chemicals that pass an electrical impulse from one neuron to another across a synapse.

non-defensiveness: Remaining calm and assertive when confronted.

nonmaleficence Do no harm; the benefit of treatment must clearly outweigh the risk of harm.

objectivity Empathy combined with professional behavior on behalf of the client produces the ability to act in the best interests of the client, even if the client does not understand or appreciate it.

obsessive-compulsive disorder Involves obsessive, unwanted, and uncontrollable thoughts, impulses, or images that intrude over and over again and override normal thoughts and actions; and a compulsive, overpowering drive to perform a set of behaviors over and over again. This compulsive behavior is a ritual intended to bring relief from the obsessive thoughts, but it can become so time-consuming as to dominate the person's life and can become a source of anxiety itself.

openness to experience One of the "big 5" personality traits openness to experience distinguishes conventional from unconventional thinking. People who are open tend to be curious, imaginative, flexible, individualistic, nonconforming, and often artistic. Closed thinking is conservative and resists change, preferring the familiar and regarding the arts and sciences as having little practical use.

organic mental disorders Temporary or permanent dysfunctions of brain tissue caused by chemicals or diseases.

pain syndrome Chronic and worsening pain in the absence of physical causes. It is self-sustaining pain that gets worse over time until it becomes chronic and debilitating. It may be started initially by acute physical pain or by emotional oversensitivity to normal discomfort, but it transforms into real pain maintained and worsened by anxiety, without any physical explanation.

panic attack A period of intense fear or discomfort in which four or more of the following symptoms are present: pounding heart, sweating, trembling, shortness of breath, feelings of choking, chest pain, nausea, feeling dizzy, and fear of losing control or dying.

panic disorder Characterized by recurrent and unexpected panic attacks. The person becomes so worried about having another attack that this intense worrying interferes with normal functioning.

paranoid personality disorder A consistent pattern of mistrust and suspicion and the perception that others have sinister intentions.

paranoid schizophrenia An affected person may hear voices telling them to do things, or have delusions of being a very important person, or of being hunted or persecuted.

parasympathetic division of the autonomic nervous system Motor neurons that conduct impulses that return the functions of the endocrine glands, heart, organs, and blood vessels back to normal.

parent The person or people who provide primary care for the child. A person may become a parent by biology, marriage, foster care, adoption, or just by being there.

parenting style Created by personality characteristics, history, current situation, and beliefs. Each parenting style is defined by the kind of interactions the parent most often has with the child.

partial loss For example, illness or disability that takes away some portion of functioning, or a divorce that reduces us to being with our children on alternate weekends and holidays.

passive aggression An action intended to harm another either physically or emotionally that is carried out with an effort to conceal the aggressor so as to avoid taking responsibility.

patient's rights Based on the concept of autonomy, which is the right to self-determination and which is ensured by the practice of informed consent.

payment-centered medical care Complex regulatory codes that attempt to balance client's rights laws with strict adherence to medical protocol in order to avoid lawsuits and insurance payment limitations to contain costs.

peripheral nervous system All the nervous tissue outside of the brain and spinal cord.

permanent loss Loss with no hope of recovery.

personal discrimination Personally denying another's access to goods, services, or opportunities based on bias.

personality A set of traits that stay the same over time and from one situation to the next.

personality development Our DNA provides plans for each personality trait. The environment determines the final expression of those genetic plans as the child moves through the stages of physical and emotional development.

personality disorders Sets of enduring traits that shape behaviors that seriously impair functioning or cause severe distress in a person's personal and social life.

personality traits with their opposites Extraversion and introversion; neuroticism and emotional stability; openness to experience and closed thinking; agreeableness and disagreeableness; and conscientiousness and impulsiveness.

phobia An abnormally fearful response to a danger that is imagined or is irrationally exaggerated.

physical boundaries Regard touch. As much as is possible, touch clients only with their permission and always touch only when it is appropriate.

physical stigma A physical imperfection that lowers a person's status within the group. This may include appearance, as well as disability and disease.

posttraumatic stress disorder (PTSD) An anxiety disorder caused by a life-threatening event or series of events that shatter an individual's sense of being able to control a situation and stay safe and secure. The threat is usually to the person themselves, but may be to someone he or she cares for deeply. Following the event or events, people have persistent flashbacks, often triggered by people, places, or events that are emotionally charged for them, in which they re-experience the original trauma. These flashbacks are so terrifying that individuals with PTSD live in fear, and construct their lives around trying to avoid anything that might trigger them, and around trying to avoid risk altogether.

prejudice Prejudging a person based on stereotyping. The assumption that a stigma tells you all you need to know to judge someone.

primary loss The initial loss. It may be either internal or external, as with a sudden heart attack or the loss of a job.

privacy Clients have the right to privacy. Some necessary conversations and procedures invade the client's privacy, but these are always performed with the client's knowledge and permission and always in as private a setting as possible. People not directly involved in and necessary to the procedure should not be there without the expressed approval of the client.

probability A predictable pattern that describes the odds of how one individual will respond to a specific parenting style.

problem solving A process that focuses on finding a solution to a problem.

professional Someone who is skilled and who is paid to apply that skill for the benefit of another.

professional relationship Exists when the professional is paid to perform their skill as a personal service for the benefit of another person.

professionalism Acting in the best interests of the client and it is a commitment to deliver quality health care to all. That commitment is honored not in spite of the negative judgments we make of some clients, but because we do not make those judgments in the first place.

profoundly mentally retarded With IQs from 20 to 40, these individuals are limited in their ability to acquire the skills necessary to take care of their personal needs, and they require supervision throughout their lives.

proposed psychological model The model proposed begins with the unconscious part of the brain detecting a lack of some element necessary for an individual to survive, develop friendships and associations, mate, protect and nurture their young, or to be fully themselves. This lack is a need and it is communicated to the conscious part of the brain by way of neurotransmitters that create a feeling. The individual processes this feeling along with other information such as the who, what, when, and where of the situation, established beliefs about self and others, and probable outcomes of various actions. These are encapsulated into self-talk, which changes the feeling into an emotion. The emotion powers an action. Together, the emotion and action comprise a behavior. The goal of the behavior is to supply the element necessary to relieve the original lack and meet the need, enabling the individual to survive, develop friendships and associations, mate, protect and nurture their young, or to be true to their own nature.

provider responsibilities The responsibilities of the provider include beneficence and nonmaleficence.

psychological dysfunction A failure of some step in the psychological functioning process that prevents a person from getting their needs met. The most common dysfunctions involve mental illness, irrational beliefs, or an inability to adjust to changes in the environment (adjustment issues).

psychological model A theoretical construct used to describe, explain, and predict psychological functioning.

quantum consciousness An emerging view of consciousness as awareness based in quantum waves isolated in the neurons of the brain. Quantum consciousness contains elements of both spiritual and chemical consciousness.

range of experience The number and variety of experiences we have had. The more experiences we have had and the more diverse those experiences have been the greater is the probability that they have challenged our beliefs and forced us to adjust.

rational beliefs Functional, as they lead to positive self-talk that promotes adjustment.

relaxation The ability to let go of everything and focus completely on what needs to be done now by learning to relax, not just the body, but the mind as well.

religion Identifies metaphysics as an existence and a power *who* creates and sustains the universe.

reptilian complex The layer of the brain immediately over the brain stem, the reptilian complex enables more complicated behavior by establishing our perception of our status (our position relative to others) and how we interact with others based on that perception.

response The reaction of some element in the territory to a behavior. It is what the person gains from the behavior. If a behavior is successful, the response meets the need that drove the behavior.

retrograde amnesia Affects the person's ability to remember things that happened before the onset of the disease. New memories are formed, but life seems to have begun at the onset of the disease.

ritual Words, tone of voice, gestures, and body language instinctively used to defend territory or status against intrusion by someone who is seen as not belonging in the territory or deserving of the status.

safety and security Come from knowing what to do. If we have no doubts about our ability to meet our physical needs, stay safe and secure, give and receive love, be accepted, and respected, we are secure and comfortable in our surroundings. For this reason, as adults we have a strong tendency to recreate the world of our childhood, maintaining the culture, position, and parenting styles we are familiar with, and seeking interaction, intimacy, and friendship with those who believe and behave in ways that make sense to us.

schizophrenia A serious mental disorder that produces symptoms that interfere with personal or social functioning for at least six months. The symptoms may include delusions, hallucinations, decreased emotional expression, disorganized speech, or disorganized behavior. Schizophrenia is separated into two types depending on whether the symptoms are positive—distortions of normal functioning, such as delusions and hallucinations, with a good chance of recovery; or negative—a loss of normal functioning, such as dulled emotions with little desire to speak or act, from which there is little chance of recovery.

schizotypical personality disorder A consistent pattern of deep mistrust of others and extreme anxiety in close relationships caused by distorted thinking and an inability to communicate. Those with this disorder view themselves as different, sometimes magical; isolated from others. This isolation becomes increasingly painful as they disengage more and more from the world around them.

science Identifies metaphysics as an existence and a power *which* creates and sustains the universe.

secondary loss Comes as a result of a primary loss; for example, a heart attack can result in the loss of employment, home, independence, feelings of self-worth, and so on.

self-talk Thoughts that continually emerge from our appraisal of each situation as we move through our day.

sensorimotor Cognitive stage from 0 to 2 years. Feelings created by sensory input (hunger, cold, etc.) lead directly to motor (physical) responses, with little complex processing.

sensory neurons A sensory neuron begins with a receptor somewhere in the body. The receptor is a switch that can be turned on by a change in the environment. When the switch is turned on an electrical current (impulse) travels through the sensory neuron and into the brain or spinal cord, where it sends neurotransmitters through a synapse to an association neuron.

separations Between people begin with differences in genetic predispositions but are magnified by the beliefs and behaviors taught by parents, status, and culture.

signs Differences that can be objectively measured, such as temperature or blood pressure, and that can be identified without the patient's participation.

skills Providing care for others involves behaviors that must be learned. Each health care specialty has its own specific skill set, but there are also skill areas that are helpful in every specialty because they are helpful in dealing with people in general, and with the stresses involved in caregiving.

social beings Humans are social beings; many needs can only be met through relationships with others.

somatic Motor neurons that carry electrical impulses to voluntary muscles, muscle that can be moved at will.

spirit Historically, consciousness has been explained as the spirit living within us.

stages of grief Denial, anger, bargaining, depression, and acceptance.

state regulations Govern the actual practice of medicine with professional practices acts that apply to the activities of hospitals, nursing homes, Medicaid programs, and medical professionals within the state.

status The person with the better territory, or more power within a mutual territory, has the higher status. They are afforded more rights and liberties and are sought after and deferred to.

stereotyping The belief that everyone who shares a specific stigma has the same character.

stigma Anything that marks a person as being different in a way that makes them lesser.

stimulus What comes just before a behavior and sets it up. It is provided by the setting the behavior takes place in. It is who, what, when, and where.

stimulus-response The nervous system allows us to recognize what is going on in the world around us and to respond to it.

stress A situation for which a substantial increase in effort is required to respond.

stress effects If we have overcome dysfunction in our life by putting in the time and effort to build new, more productive pathways we must always be aware that stress can drive us back to using the old, dysfunctional ones. When under significant stress it is of the utmost importance that we just do not act. We cannot resolve conflicts, discipline our child, or make important decisions. In this condition the last thing we may want to do is stop and walk away, but anything we do will most likely only make things worse. There will be another day, and we can address issues on that day without the risk of hurting those we love or destroying our worlds.

stress reaction A set of predictable stages that develop in response to unrelieved stress.

structural divisions of the brain Structurally, the brain is divided into the brain stem, the diencephalon, the cerebellum, and the cerebrum.

sudden loss Could be an unexpected accident, heart attack, or layoff. Sudden loss gives no time for preparation and can present severe grief and be an acute challenge to one's coping ability.

summation The total effect of all of the neurotransmitters and neuroinhibitors sent from all of the other neurons with which one neuron is connected. If the neurotransmitters received outnumber the neuroinhibitors received by a large enough margin an electrical impulse is generated.

supportive parenting Involves making and consistently enforcing rules in the best interests of the child, as with assertive parenting; but with supportive parenting the child is always included in making the rules and can always question a decision after it is made, provided that the questioning is done in an appropriate manner.

suppressed grief Grief is repressed, unfelt perhaps for years, but some future event may unexpectedly trigger its release.

symbolic functions Cognitive stage from 2 to 7 years. The ability to create and maintain mental images and symbols and to express them as language develops rapidly. Children learn and use self-advancing bargains and compromises to stay safe and secure and to get what they want or avoid what they don't want.

sympathetic division of the autonomic nervous system Motor neurons that conduct impulses that move the functioning of the endocrine glands, heart, organs, and blood vessels away from normal. The sympathetic division is responsible for fight-or-flight and stress reactions.

symptoms Differences that are subjectively experienced, such as dizziness or pain; they are felt by the patient but cannot be seen by the doctor.

synapse A specialized structure that forms a junction between two neurons or between a neuron and another type of cell. This structure uses chemicals called neurotransmitters to pass an electrical impulse across a gap from one cell to the next. A neuron usually has thousands and sometimes more than a hundred thousand connections with other neurons.

temporary loss Loss with good hope of recovery.

territory The people, places, and things people depend on to meet their needs; it may include family, friends, home, job, career, achievements, and reputation.

them Those we do not recognize as belonging in our territory or at our level of status and who are not accepted or allowed.

therapeutic relationship A relationship that helps a person to heal. It enhances the quality of life by encouraging acceptance and hope; supporting effort and activity; and focusing on what can be accomplished.

total loss For example, the death of a loved one, or learning that one has a terminal disease.

tracts Long bundles of nerve fibers that carry electrical impulses inside of the central nervous system.

traumatic amnesia It is usually due to a head injury. Depending on the severity of the injury it may be temporary or permanent and it may be retrograde, anterograde, or both.

tribal stigma A mark or quality that identifies a person as belonging to another group. This may include things such as color, religion, language, accent, clothing, and economic level.

uncertain loss Some diseases, such as multiple sclerosis, have a high degree of uncertainty. It can never be known when a remission will give way to a renewed onslaught of the disease or how much or what kind of damage may be done during an acute phase. The person must be able to live with the uncertainty and cope with the losses as they occur.

us Those we recognize as belonging in our territory and who are accepted and allowed.

us versus them Others who are not from my world can be relegated to the fringes of humanity; they can become "them" while we are "us."

void The metaphysical realm beyond time and space which created and sustains the universe.

wait Avoiding the natural impulse to make snap judgments of others and taking the time needed to form a broader, more realistic appraisal.

Bibliography

American Psychiatric Association. (1994). *Diagnostic and statistical manual of mental disorders* (4th ed.). Washington, DC.: American Psychiatric Association.

American Psychiatric Association. (2000). *Diagnostic and statistical manual IV—text revision* (4th ed.). Washington, DC.: American Psychiatric Association.

Aurell, Carl G. (1983). Perception: a model comprising two modes of consciousness. Addendum: Evidence based on event-related potentials and brain lesions. *Perceptual and motor skills, 56,* 211–220.

Bargh, J. A. (1994). The four horsemen of automaticity: Awareness, intention, efficiency, and control in social cognition. In R. S. Wyer, Jr., & T. K. Srull (Eds.), *Handbook of social cognition* (2nd ed., Vol. 1, pp. 1–40). Hillsdale, NJ: Erlbaum.

Bouchard, T. J., Jr. (1994). Genes, environment, and personality. *Science, 264,* 1700–1701.

Bouchard, T. J., Jr., Lykken, D. T., McGue, M., Segal, N. L., & Tellegen, A. (1990). Sources of human psychological differences: The Minnesota study of twins reared apart. *Science, 250,* 223–228.

Brewer, M. (1979). In-group bias in the minimal intergroup situation: A cognitive motivational analysis. *Psychological Bulletin, 86,* 307–324.

Brown, W. A. (1997). The placebo effect. *Scientific American,* 90–95.

Caplan, G. (1990). Loss, stress, and mental health. *Community mental health journal, 26*(1), 27–48.

Cassel, E. J. (2000). The principles of the Belmont Report revisited: How have respect for persons, beneficence and justice been applied to clinical medicine? *Hastings Center Report, 30*(4), 12–21.

Chapman, K. J., & Pepler, C. (1998). Coping, hoping, and anticipatory grief in family members in palliative home care. *Cancer Nursing, 21*(4), 226–234.

Cornell-Bell, A. H., Finkbeiner, S. M. (1991). Ca^{2+} waves in astrocytes. *Cell Calcium, 12,* 185–204.

Cornell-Bell, A. H., Finkbeiner, S. M., Cooper, M. S., & Smith, S. J. (1990). Glutamate induces calcium waves in cultured astrocytes: long-range glial signaling. *Science, 247,* 470–473.

Cornell-Bell, A. H., Thomas, P. G., Caffrey, J. M. (1992). Ca^{2+} and filopodial responses to glutamate in cultured astrocytes and neurons. *Canadian Journal of Physiology and Pharmacologyl, 70,* S206–S218.

Cunningham, W. E., Burton, T. M., Hawes-Dawson, J., Kington, R. S., & Hays, R. D. (2000). Use of relevancy ratings by target respondents to develop health-related quality of life measures: An example with African-American elderly. *Quality of Life Research, 8,* 749–768.

Diamond, M. C., Law, F., Rhodes, H., Linder, B., Rosenzweig, M. R., Krech, D., & Bennett, E. L. (1966). Increases in cortical depth and glia numbers in rats subjected to enriched environments. *Comparative Neurology, 128,* 117–126.

Drench, M. E., Noonan, A. C., Sharby, N., Hallenborg Ventura, S., (2003). *Psychosocial Aspects of Health Care* (pp. 256–257). New Jersey: Prentice Hall.

Egan, T. (1999). In the war against drugs, treatment is proving a winner. *San Diego Union-Tribune,* E14.

Erikson, E. H. (1963). *Childhood and society.* New York: Norton.

Erikson, E. H. (1982). *The life cycle completed*: Review. New York: Norton.

Erlin, J. A. (1998). Culture, ethics, and respect: The bottom line is understanding. *Orthopaedic Nursing, 17*(6), 79–82.

Esler, J. L., & Bock, B. C. (2004). Psychological treatments for noncardiac chest pain: Recommendation for a new approach. *Journal of Psychosomatic Research, 56,* 263–269.

Fields, H. L., & Basbaum, A. (1999). Central nervous system mechanisms of pain modulation. In P. D. Wall and R. Melzak (Eds.), *Textbook of Pain* (4th ed., pp. 309–328). New York: Churchill Livingstone.

Forward, S. (1989). *Toxic Parents.* New York: Bantam Books.

Frankl, V. E. (1984). *Man's search for meaning: An introduction to logotherapy* (3rd ed.). New York: Simon & Schuster.

Friedman, M. (1997). Post-traumatic stress disorder. *Journal of Clinical Psychiatry, 58*(Suppl. 9), 33–36.

Gardner, H. (1993). *Multiple intelligences: The theory in practice* (p. 254). New York: Basic Books.

Gilliland, G., & Fleming, S. (1998). A comparison of spousal anticipatory grief and conventional grief. *Death Studies, 22*(6), 541–569.

Glod, C. (1998). *Contemporary psychiatric-mental health nursing.* Philadelphia: F. A. Davis.

Greenough, W. T., Volkmar, F. R., & Juraska, J. M. (1973). Effects of rearing complexity on dendritic branching in frontolateral and temporal cortex of the rat. *Experimental Neurology, 41,* 371–378.

Greenwald, A. G., & Banaji, M. R. (1995). Implicit social cognition: Attitudes, self esteem and stereotypes: More evidence for the role of affect in health care. *Health Psychology, 12*(2), 140–146.

Greenwald, A. G., & Banaji, M. R. (1995). Implicit social cognition: Attitudes, self esteem and stereotypes. *Psychological Review, 102*(1), 4–27.

Grigorenko, E. L. (2000). Heritability and intelligence. In R. J. Sternberg, *Handbook of intelligence.* New York: Cambridge University Press.

Hanson, G., & Venturelli, P. J. (1998). *Drugs and Society* (5th ed.). Boston: Jones and Barlett.

Howell, D., Butler, L., Vincent, L., Watt-Watson, J., & Stearns, N. (2000). Influencing nurses' knowledge, attitudes, and practice in cancer pain management. *Cancer Nursing, 23*(1), 55–63.

Huttenlocker, P. R. (1994). Synaptogenesis in human cerebral cortex. In G. Dawson & K. W. Fischer (Eds.), *Human behavior and the Developing Brain* (pp. 35–54). New York: Guilford.

John, O. P., & Srivastava, S. (1999). The big five trait taxonomy: History, measurement and theoretical perspectives. In L. A. Pervin & O. P. John (Eds.),

Handbook of personality (2nd ed.). New York: Guilford.

Kasar, J., & Clark, E. N. (2000). *Developing professional behaviors.* Thorofare, NJ: Slack.

Kohlberg, L. (1984). *The psychology of moral development: Essays on moral development* (Vol. 11). San Francisco: Harper & Row.

Kuan, C.-Y., Roth, K. A., Flavell, R. A., & Rakic, P. (2000). Mechanisms of programmed cell death in the developing brain. *Trends in Neuroscience, 23,* 291–297.

Kubler-Ross, E. (1969). *On death and dying.* New York: Macmillan.

Lauder, J. M. (1998). Neurotransmitters as morphogens. *Progress in Brain Research, 73,* 365–388.

Leo, J. (1987, January 12). Exploring the traits of twins. *Time.*

Lewin, R. (1974, October 5). Observing the Brain Through a Cat's Eyes. *Saturday Review/World.*

Maslow, A. H. (1970). *Motivation and personality* (2nd ed.). New York: Harper & Row.

McCullough, M. E., Bellah, C. G., Kilpatrick, S. D., & Johnson, J. L. (2001). Vengefulness: Relationships with forgiveness, rumination, well being, and the Big Five. *Personality and Social Psychology Bulletin, 27,* 601–610.

Melzack, R., & Wall, P. D. (1965). Pain mechanisms: A new theory. *Science, 150,* 971–979.

Mindell, A. (2000). *Quantum mind.* Portland, OR: Lao Tse Press. Social interaction and brain development.

Nagi, S. (1965). Some conceptual issues in disability and rehabilitation. In M. Sussman (Ed.), *Sociology and Rehabilitation* (pp. 100–113). Washington, DC: American Sociological Association.

Operario, D., & Fiske, S. T. (2001). Stereotypes: Content, structures, processes, and context. In R. Brown & S. L. Gaertner (Eds.), *Blackwell handbook of social psychology: Interpersonal processes.* Malden, MA: Blackwell.

Perry, B. D. (1994). Neurobiological sequelae of childhood trauma: Post traumatic stress disorders in children. In M. Murberg (Ed.), *Catecholamines in Post Traumatic Stress Disorder: Emerging Concepts* (pp. 253–276). Washington, DC.: American Psychiatric Press.

Perry, B. D., & Pollard, R. (1998). Homeostasis, stress, trauma, and adaptation: A neurodevelopmental view of childhood trauma. *Child and Adolescent Psychiatric Clinics of North America, 7,* 33–51.

Peters, S. A., Palay, S. L., Webster, H. (1991). *The neuroglial cells.* In *The Fine Structure of the Nervous System: Neurons and Their Supporting Cells* (pp. 273–295). London: Oxford Press.

Rakic, P. (1981). Development of cerebral centers in the primate brain depends on binocular competition before birth. *Science, 214,* 928–931.

Rakic, P. (1996). Development of the cerebral cortex in human and non-human primates. In M. Lewis (Ed.), *Child and Adolescent Psychiatry: A Comprehensive Textbook* (pp. 9–30). New York: Williams and Wilkins.

Roth, D., Slone, M., & Dar, R. (2000). Which way cognitive development? *Theory and Psychology, 10,* 353–373.

Sagan, C. (1977). *The Dragons of Eden.* New York: Ballantine Books.

Salkovskis, P. M. (1992, May 27). Psychological Treatment of Noncardiac Chest Pain: The Cognitive Approach. *The American Journal of Medicine, Vol. 92.*

Schuckit, M. A. (2000). *Drug and alcohol abuse* (5th ed.). New York: Kluwer Academic.

Seroka, A. M. (1994). Values clarification and ethical decision-making. *Seminars for Nurse Managers, 2*(1), 8–15.

Siegler, M. A. (2000). Professional values in modern clinical practice. *Hastings Center report, 30*(4), S19–S22.

Silverstone, P. (1996). Prevalence of psychiatric disorders in medical patients. *Journal of Nervous and Mental Diseases, 84*(1), 43–50.

Sulmasy, D. P. (1997). *The healer's calling.* Mahwah, NJ: Paulist Press.

Surgeon General's call to action to prevent suicide. (1999). Retrieved from: http://www.surgeongeneral. gov/osg/calltoaction.

Swick, H. M. (1998). Academic medicine must deal with the clash of business and professional values. *Academic medicine, 73*(7), 751–755.

Sylwester, R. (1997). *Windows to the mind, Volume 1.* Tuscon, AZ: Zephyr Press.

Talbot, M. (2000, January 9). The placebo prescription. *New York Times Magazine,* p. 34. (Vargha-Khadem, F. (2000, November 20). Cited in J. Fischman, Seeds of a sociopath. *U.S. News & World Report,* p. 82.

Waddell, G. (1987). A new clinical model for the treatment of low back pain. *Spine, 12*(7), 632–644.

Weiner, B. (1980). A cognitive (attribution)-emotion-action model of motivated behavior: An analysis of judgments of help-giving. *Journal of Personality and Social Psychology, 39*(2), 186–200.

Weisman, A. (1998). The patient with acute grief. In T. Stern, J. Herman, & J. Slavin (Eds.), *The Massachusetts General Hospital (MGH) guide to psychiatry in primary care* (pp. 25–31). New York: McGraw-Hill.

Weissberg, M. (1999). Cognitive aspects of pain. In P. D. Wall and R. Melzak (Eds.), *Textbook of Pain* (4th ed., pp. 345–358). New York: Churchill Livingstone.

Wiggins, J. S., & Trapnell, P. D. (1997). Personality structure: The return of the big five. In R. Hogan, J. Johnson, & S. Briggs (Eds.), *Handbook of personality psychology.* San Diego, CA: Academic Press.

Wise, M. G., Gray, K. F., & Seltzer, B. (1999). Delerium, Dementia, and amnestic disorders. In R. E. Hales, S. C. Yudofsky, & J. A. Talbott (Eds.), *The American Psychiatric Press textbook of psychiatry* (3rd ed., pp 317–362). Washington, DC: American Psychiatric Press.

World Health Organization. (2000). About WHO: Definition of Health. In *World Health Organization.* Retrieved from: http://www.who. int/aboutwho/en/definition.html Weissberg, 1999).

Index